New Cancer Thera

New Cancer Therapies

The Patient's Dilemma

Penelope Williams

FIREFLY BOOKS

A FIREFLY BOOK

Published by Firefly Books Ltd. 2000

First Printing

U.S. CATALOGING IN PUBLICATION DATA

Williams, Penelope
        New cancer therapies: the patient's dilemma
Penelope Williams.—1st ed.
[328] p. : cm. – (Your Personal Health)
Includes index.
Summary: The issues cancer patients face after diagnosis, particularly in the context of alternative and conventional treatments.
ISBN 1-55209-485-5
1.   Cancer—Alternative treatment. 2. Cancer–
Treatment. 3. Cancer–Popular works. I. Title.
II. Series
616.99406 -dc21   2000   CIP

Published in the United States in 2000 by
Firefly Books (U.S.) Inc.
P.O. Box 1338, Ellicott Station
Buffalo, New York, USA
14205

Published in Canada in 2000 by Key Porter Books Limited.

Electronic formatting: Heidi Palfrey
Design: Peter Maher

Printed and bound in Canada

Great is the power of steady misrepresentation.

Charles Darwin, *On the Origin of Species*,
introduction to the 1872 edition

Acknowledgments

First, I want to thank all of the cancer patients who were willing to take the time to tell me their stories. For many, this meant carving precious moments out of lives that had little time left to share. Theirs is an unequaled courage and generosity of spirit.

My thanks, too, to the doctors and researchers who explained medical issues and gave me the view from the other side of cancer. In this group are those who preferred to remain anonymous because of their concern that any association with alternative cancer therapies might hurt their career in the medical mainstream.

I am particularly grateful to all the staff at the IAT Clinic in the Bahamas for their cooperation and openness, especially Dr. John Clement, Edmund Granger, Lynn Austin, and June Austin. Their friendly help and generous giving of their time always made me feel so welcome.

To all those who have helped me from the earliest days, many thanks—Sally Armstrong who published my article on alternative therapies in *Homemaker's* magazine, and then said, write a book about these people, these issues; Jennifer Barclay who so enthusiastically supported the idea; Susan Renouf who was willing to take a risk; Barbara Berson who gave me such wise and intelligent editorial guidance; Ainsley Spry who spent hours transcribing tapes and illegible interview notes; Andrea Spry who asked the tough questions; Loranne Sackmann-Meloche who fought so hard for a friend's right to make treatment choices; Sharon Batt who so generously shared her own research; Carol Burnham Cook at Willow, and the librarians at the Beattie Cancer Library who tracked down elusive quotes, facts, and statistics; Dianne Perrier who helped guide PMF during my many absences from the office; Pat Hood who helped create the index in jig-time; and the Ontario Arts Program for a writer's reserve grant.

And finally, my special thanks and gratitude to Allen Sackmann, my husband, front-line editor, sounding board, devil's advocate, and supporter, and as ever, and always, to my sons Sam and Matt for their constant encouragement and steadfast faith in my endeavors.

Contents

Introduction

Let me be absolutely clear. This book is about cancer, cancer patients, and the issues they face after diagnosis. It is not a tirade against establishment medicine or a paean of praise for all alternative cancer therapies. However, it does put the latter into the realm of realistic options and pleads for a fair hearing. In the present climate, that is asking a lot.

In the current state of cancer treatment, patients rarely have the dubious luxury of concentrating solely on their disease. Cancer not only comes cloaked in horrific images of madly multiplying cells and suppurating tumors; it also trails a bewildering array of issues. There are medical turf wars, conspiracy theories, conflicting research, and shifting statistics; announcements and denouncements of cures; risk factors that change like chameleons; debates on patients' rights and responsibilities; arguments about the accuracy, efficacy, and ethics of clinical trials; disagreement among practitioners and among treatment centers; and second, third, and fourth opinions on everything. For many patients, the most contentious debate—the widest schism of all—is that between conventional and alternative approaches to cancer treatment. For those caught in cancer's maw, the disputation around these issues is not distant thunder. It is a loud roaring amplified by their impending mortality.

Discussions of cancer therapies usually support one of the two approaches: conventional (see also "industrialized" and "establishment") versus non-conventional (see also "unconventional," "alternative," and "unproven"). Rarely do you see them joined by "and." A communication fault line bites right through the middle, ensuring that the chasm between the two remains deep. Throughout the history of medicine it has been ever thus.

During the four years of researching and writing this book I have been struck again and again by just how wide that chasm is. For many, the very existence of the field of alternative cancer therapies is an affront. However, its existence also underlines one inescapable fact: conventional treatments are not winning the war against cancer.

This book had its genesis in a magazine article I wrote in October 1995. Entitled "Cancer: New Frontiers," it discussed alternative therapies and offered a gentle plea for cessation of hostilities between the two camps. There were lots of letters in response, both positive and negative. But one in particular I remember, from a doctor who was incensed that I had had the temerity to write about the subject at all.

A discussion of cancer treatments seems to produce knee-jerk responses to criticism of either approach. People form up into opposing camps, and the middle ground disappears under a carpet of misinformation and emotion. The first casualty is facts; the second is reasonable discussion; but the most serious casualties of all are people with cancer who must slog through the mud flung by both sides, motivated not by the challenge of a lively debate but by the goal of achieving their own survival.

Why is the subject so controversial? At a dinner party of old and good friends, the subject of alternative therapies came up. In less than a minute we were at it, hammer and tongs.

"Listen to what I am saying, not what you think you hear me saying," I kept repeating ever more quietly, finally in an astonished whisper. My plea that other approaches to cancer treatment be given a fair hearing was interpreted as total endorsement of anything alternative. A comment on the failure of chemotherapy in treating a specific cancer was translated into a blanket condemnation of all conventional treatments. And such criticism seemed to be considered as outrageous as an attack on motherhood. Chemotherapy is not motherhood. Radiation is not motherhood. What was the problem here? Why were we all so emotional about the subject?

You'd be hard pressed to find anyone in our society who has not been scorched by the fiery breath of cancer, either directly or when a family member, friend, or co-worker is diagnosed or dies. This is not just because of an aging population, although that is part of it. As one friend said that night, "If you had asked us to list our values by priority twenty years ago, health would not have been up there. Now it's at the top."

The incidence of cancer overall is climbing; for some specific ones, such as prostate cancer, and lung cancer among women, the increase is precipitous, the graph lines nearly perpendicular. Between 1969 and 1989 in Canada, the incidence of cancer increased by more than 100 percent. (And these numbers do not include the enormous jump in the incidence of skin cancer.) In 1999, it is estimated that there will be 129,300 new cases of cancer and 63,400 deaths from the disease (National Cancer Institute of Canada, 1999). In the United States, cancer statistics paint an equally grim picture. In 1997, 539,577 people died of this disease, making it the second highest cause of death in that country (CDC, 1999).

However, these statistics alone do not explain the touchiness of the topic. Add to the mix the weekly media announcements of new cancer cures that somehow never arrive on the street. Patients go to their doctors clutching a clipping of the latest breakthrough only to be told that it's not really anything new, it's not yet available, it's still in trials and will be for several years, it only works in mice, it doesn't work at all. . . .

Juxtapose the Good News media clamor with the indisputable fact that people are dying of this "curable" disease every day. It is understandable to me that patients are beginning to look further afield for a way of arresting the disease rampant within them. But not to everyone, apparently. When hundreds of cancer patients and their families flocked to hear Dr. Luigi di Bella from Italy explain his alternative approach to cancer treatment, Dr. Andrew Arnold, one of the team of Canadian doctors studying Dr. di Bella's procedures, termed the huge interest "very meddlesome" ("Cancer Doctor a Superstar," *Ottawa Citizen*, June 8, 1998).

When thirteen-year-old Tyrell Dueck and his parents decided against any more chemotherapy to treat his cancer, opting to leave Saskatchewan to try an alternative approach at a Mexican cancer clinic, they incurred the wrath not only of the medical establishment but of the courts as well. The Duecks were not granted freedom of choice until the Canadian doctors deemed that his cancer had spread too far for it to matter what treatment they chose.

It is difficult for conventional cancer specialists when patients turn away from them to try something else. Many see only that patients are undermining their chances for recovery by chasing "will-o'-the-wisp" cures. But it is even harder for most patients. To go against the medical status quo is a lonely and frightening undertaking, especially when lives are at stake—their own. Adding volatility to the mix are the anxiety and anger both of people who question an institution they have been raised to accept as sacrosanct and also of those who defend it. Even if a patient simply asks if there is anything beyond radiation, surgery, and chemotherapy, many doctors see the question as a personal affront. This is hard on doctors, no question. It is also hard on patients when they see not only their health but their doctors' authority undermined by a disease that defies conventional ministrations.

The mix of issues and the atmosphere of hostility and miscommunication mean that few physicians and healers from either camp are willing to listen, to share, and to work together toward the common goal of curing cancer, never mind how we get there. Unfortunately, the end does not appear to justify the means here.

I come to this subject not just as a researcher and writer but as someone who has been there—indeed, in a sense, who is still there. Following a diagnosis of breast cancer in late 1988, I had surgery, chemotherapy, and radiation, a year of treatment affectionately known as "Slash, Poison and Burn." Somewhere about the third month of chemotherapy, I started to think—with what brain cells I had salvaged from the engulfing terror of a cancer diagnosis—that there had to be a better way. Why, in these days of modern medicine, was the treatment for cancer almost as bad as the disease? This questioning continues to be reinforced. Recently a friend told me that her doctors had recommended a double prophylactic mastectomy because she was in a high-risk category for recurrence of her breast cancer. In the same evening, a young man told me of his wife's fight against breast cancer. Bone-marrow transplantation bought her a few months, but when the cancer metastasized to the liver, she was given Taxotere, a highly toxic chemotherapy drug. She was dead within a week. The drug had killed her before the cancer could. In a keynote speech at the First World Conference on Breast Cancer in 1997, Dr. Susan Love, author of *The Susan Love Breast Book*, predicted that in a few years we would look back with utter disbelief at the use of such medieval treatments as chemotherapy and preventative amputations. But we're not there yet.

During my own chemotherapy and radiation treatments, the cancer cells may not have multiplied but the questions did. Why did the medical establishment seem so threatened by anything beyond the three major pillars of cancer treatment? Was it really a conspiracy? Did none of these non-conventional therapies work? Just what was going on? That was eleven years ago. Some would say that the conventional approaches cured me. Others would say I have survived breast cancer, to date, despite such treatment. Some would say that attitude, hope, and motivation have kept my cancer at bay. Others would say, that's just New Age talk. There is no evidence. There are no clinical trials for attitude, hope, and motivation. I would say, I do not know. And because there is no certainty of a cure for cancer, the specter of recurrence is always lurking.

In spite of research, clinical studies, and statistics, in spite of evidence-based "proof" (deriving from controlled studies and clinical trials), empirical "proof" (deriving from general observation of results), and anecdotal "proof" (individual successes or failures), cancer still remains an enigma—its cause and its cure. Every practitioner wants to be able to say, "Do this and your cancer will be cured." Every patient wants to hear the same thing. Since this is not happening, the subject whirls in a vortex of frustration and rage. Researchers inch slowly ahead; the media leap forward; hopes are raised only to be dashed. Newspaper editorials, books, articles, television and radio documentaries, and the Internet pour out information that, when parsed with the attention sharpened by first-hand experience with the disease, falls apart. New therapies are praised and damned. Clinical studies contradict each other. And in the middle of it all are the patients who do not have the plexiglass protection of science and statistics or the luxury of time to weigh the evidence of study after study, to wait for science to find the cure. In increasing numbers, they are looking for ways beyond the conventional to fight the disease raging within their own bodies.

These are the people who will not accept the death sentence that a diagnosis of cancer at first appears to be. They arm themselves with information; knowledge of patients' rights; support from families, from organizations, from some doctors. This book is their story. Its focus is on the *personal* dilemma for cancer patients, not the *medical* debate on the success rate of specific therapies.

Many of the patients whose stories are included here I met at the Immuno-Augmentative Therapy (IAT) Clinic in Freeport, Grand Bahama. The IAT Clinic is a micro example of a macro problem—the cancer establishment's rejection of any treatment other than the three modalities of surgery, chemotherapy, and radiation. I have interviewed patients and staff at the IAT Clinic for four years, studying medical records of patients—of some who are alive and well, some who are holding their own, and some who have died; I have gathered empirical evidence of IAT's efficacy with certain cancers as well as anecdotal evidence of successes. I chose IAT because I was personally impressed by the place and the people, but also, more important for this book, because in working there I had no restrictions placed on me, no barriers raised, no public relations "spins" imposed. Medical records were made available. Any current or former patient and patient's family member I could interview at my discretion, if they were willing. No one refused to speak to me. All but one patient from IAT wanted their real names to be used. The one who didn't was afraid that his doctor back home would find out that he had strayed from the conventional path and would refuse to treat him.

I am not claiming that IAT is the magic bullet that is going to cure cancer. The medical staff at IAT do not make that claim either. However, although IAT *is* an example of a therapy beyond the conventional trio that deserves fair consideration, it continues to be ostracized by the cancer establishment. Although empirical data of its success in the treatment of some cancers come from patient case histories and not from the formal construct of clinical trials, they present a picture of a viable cancer treatment. The IAT story focuses all the issues—evidence-based medicine versus empirical-based; treatment of a person versus treatment of a disease; cost; the power of the status quo; turf wars—and, most important of all, the experience of the cancer patient in each world.

The history of medicine is the backdrop, *plus ça change, plus c'est la même chose*—the status quo is so hard to shift, and has been since the time of Hippocrates. Surgeons were barbers until they scrambled up to the top of the mountain. Oncologists were poisoners, radiologists were murderers. The kings of the peak now defend their territory with "science"—therapies tested by the rules of the scientific method—to the exclusion of all other approaches. But alternative therapists (so named only because they provide an alternative to the mainstream of the moment; some therapies now deemed "alternative" *were* the mainstream centuries ago)—including the immunologists, the geneticists, and the practitioners of eastern medicine—are inching up the mountain.

Common threads stitch the quilt of the patients' experiences described here, not just those of people who have gone and continue to go to the IAT Clinic, but all the stories: the harsh statistics indicating little progress in the conventional war against cancer; the incredible power of hope, so often poleaxed by statistics; and the crazy dance of researchers, politicians, medical experts and, sadly, patients themselves, at the altar of the many cancers for which we have no cure. Because we do not know what causes that first cell to run amok, we spin out a host of possibilities that might stop its course. This arsenal includes the conventional Big Guns—of surgery, radiation, and chemotherapy—fired and guided by clinical studies and statistics; the kinder, gentler weapons of immunology and hormone therapies; as well as the holistic treatments, the mind/body approaches, diet, herbs, tinctures, and prayer. And we all dance to the beat of the latest risk factors, which change with the latest headline. In the face of all this, doesn't it make sense for researchers, regulators, and physicians to work together, to stop defending the status quo with such ferocity, and to concentrate their energy on defeating the disease itself?

1

Cancer Diagnosis: Passport to Another Place

Pick a day, any day. It will be a date seared on the heart and mind of someone—many someones—who learned that day that she or he has cancer. The disease arrives in lives sometimes with the suddenness of a grenade, sometimes on cat's paws, via the slow inexorable fog of symptoms and the water torture of tests, to the tentative and then final diagnosis. So often, cancer comes cloaked in another guise, lurking in a muscle or organ, disguised as something so much more benign. And so often does the treatment. Cancer therapies also come in a variety of forms, many as bewildering—a few as destructive—as the disease itself.

The date Diane will never forget is Labor Day, the first Monday in September 1996. Her nightmare began with a tingling down one side of her body that finally had to be acknowledged. Over the summer months she had ignored it, treating it as something that would just go away, as aches and pains do. It didn't. The tingling grew worse, and her doctor gave her medication for high blood pressure. The symptoms persisted, the tingling settling into numbness, a pattern that ruled out hypertension. She had a chest X-ray just before going away for the long weekend and returned to three messages from her doctor's office. She should come in immediately; something had turned up on the X-ray. The "something" was four tumors in the lung. Prognosis: "The surgeon said there was a 95 percent mortality rate with this form of lung cancer. The oncologist told me 100 percent mortality, that there was no treatment, no survival. It was not a matter of years but of months."

Swollen feet and ankles gave Dave notice that something was amiss. His wife's insistence that he go for a battery of tests, including one for hepatitis C, flipped open the starting gates. The confirmed diagnosis of liver cancer as well as hepatitis C fixed the date in his mind forever. For Dave, forever was less than two years.

In 1990, Theresa plunged into the cold ocean for an early season swim. The shock of the frigid water took her breath away, but the sense of suffocation did not abate as she warmed up. It did not abate for months. The year was well into the warm summer days of July when it was confirmed that the cause of her breathlessness was cancer.

"I was in medical books because—the only word they could use was 'humongous' to describe the tumor in my chest cavity; it had collapsed my lung, it had shoved my heart up into my shoulder; it had enlarged my heart; the tumor was wrapped around my oesophagus, it was completely inoperable. It was so advanced and so huge, they put my charts, scans, and MRIs in front of three hundred medical students and said, 'OK, what would your diagnosis be?' The consensus was 'Well, obviously, this woman didn't make it,' and then they wanted to wheel me in in a wheelchair, and I am like, 'No, please, let me walk,' and they couldn't believe that I was alive." Her lymphoma was "the most malignant there is." That early season swim launched her into the sea of cancer. She is still swimming; not drowning, but waving.

For Bill, it was a sudden pain under his shoulder blade when he sneezed. Pulled muscle, he thought. Wrong. His GP found a "fatty cyst" in his back. He cut into the flesh, but quickly closed up the wound: "I don't want to mess with this—the growth is tangled up in the muscle." The growth was not a cyst, but it was several weeks before the diagnosis was confirmed: rhabdomyosarcoma, a cancer very rarely found in adults. Bill was forty-one years old. His medical records from that date in 1993 read like a curriculum vitae written by Kafka:

- 1993—6 cm tumor removed from back
- June 1995—metastasis to lung, resected [surgery]
- February 1996—recurrence—repeat chest wall resection
- October 1996—metastasis to duodenum, surgery to remove mass
- April 1997—another lesion in duodenum; surgery

Steve's colon cancer might have gone undetected for years if he had not gone for his wife's physical: "My wife was to go for her regular annual checkup but didn't feel well, so I phoned the doctor: 'OK if I come instead of my wife?'"

After the examination, the doctor pronounced him in great shape, perfect condition for a sixty-three-year-old. "But a guy your age, you've never had a colonoscopy? You should." Within five minutes they found a tumor. Surgery revealed several more, with metastasis to the liver.

An annual physical, required by his employer's insurance company, was Paul's ticket to ride the cancer train. It was one of those appointments you pencil into your calender without much thought. An irritant, really, in a busy schedule. Go for the physical then go for a game of squash. Been doing this for years. This time it was different. At the age of forty-seven, at the peak of apparent good health, Paul was told he had colon cancer with metastases to the liver. It was January 13, 1997.

Barbara found the lump in her breast when she was nursing her baby. That was the first time around. The second time, ten years later, the discovery was heralded by a tumble from her horse. Persistent pain in the sternum was puzzling because it didn't seem connected with her fall. Red flag. A bone scan revealed that the cancer was back, not just in her sternum, but in the lumbar and thoracic spine. Three years before, a bone scan had detected nothing. What had this to do with her fall? Who knows. Recurrence, or recognition of it, apparently is triggered by all sorts of oddities. She said, "My oncologist told me, 'people tell me, "I was fine until my cat spit up on me". . . .'"

Earl fell down the stairs, and the pain in his chest—presumably from a cracked rib—would not go away. It would not go away because it was a large tumor in the lung, not a cracked rib at all. Earl's journey took him to conventional cancer centers and alternative treatment centers; he took vitamins and herbs. He changed his diet. His wife, Leslye, became his full-time care organizer and partner in his quest for prolongation and quality of life. According to his surgeon, their efforts earned him at least an extra year.

Liam was twelve years old, a kid poised on the threshold of summer, that hot, idyllic cottage time when the only worry is whether the rain will put out the campfire, the only decision whether to swim before or after playing hide-and-seek in the woods. But Liam started having headaches. The idyllic summer slowly metamorphosed into a tunnel of bedroom-dark days, sickening pain, problems with blurred vision, and finally a seizure in the hospital lab. The diagnosis was "growing pains," or maybe food allergies. His parents pushed, cajoled, threatened, and pleaded for proper tests and an end to brush-offs. Liam had a malignant brain tumor.

Sue's journey started with childhood leukemia, progressed to thyroid cancer, and blossomed into breast cancer with metastases to the liver and bones. Of her thirty-seven years, twenty-three have been laced with cancer. In November 1997 her prognosis was three months more of life. The doctors offered her yet more chemotherapy, high-dose, very toxic. Could this cure her? No. It might buy her two or three more months, "if it doesn't kill you."

All these people have more than their cancer in common; they have a determination to find a way to reclaim their lives from illness, whatever route it takes. They have all struggled in the quicksand of conflicting information, promised cures, and smashed hopes. Many, like those patients at the Immuno-Augmentative Therapy Clinic in the Bahamas, or the alternative cancer clinics in Mexico, and those who choose holistic and homeopathic physicians or who combine alternative with conventional treatments, find themselves on the road less traveled, away from the paved highways of conventional treatment. They have taken on the frightening responsibility of making personal decisions on how they and their disease should be treated, often in opposition to their medical team, their families, even the law. It is an intimidating gamble, because their lives are the poker chips.

Some patients arrive at the fork in the road very early on, the very precise delineation between the alternative and the conventional therapy routes; for others, the pathway is linear. Sue traveled along the conventional route until it petered out, then moved along the alternative course. Others, like Paul, rejected the conventional medical highway in favor of another route right from the beginning. For still others, it is Hobson's choice. Diane was faced with an alternative approach or nothing, since chemotherapy and radiation were not an option, except as palliative care.

So pick a day, any day. This time it is you to whom the doctor says, "Your test results are in and, I'm sorry to tell you, you have cancer." What now? In those three words, your old world has crashed and burned. You hear the diagnosis, and your life ends. Really, though, you are just beginning a new one, in another place, another world with a whole new set of rules and priorities. Your new world takes misty shape, a desolate and foreign landscape.

Cancer. The very word slams through your casual expectations of living forever, or at least the allotted three score years and ten. You struggle with all the baggage cancer trails with it—the chilling statistics, the graphic images of pain and decay, the despair of seeing your life spin out of control. Then, as the fog of terror begins to lift, and you cast about for a medical route that will deliver you from this nightmare, another fog rolls in, this time of conflicting information. And the terror engulfs you again. Because what if you don't make the right choice? *Is* there a right choice?

Bad enough that every book or magazine you read, every video you watch, tape you hear, or web site you visit makes claim for a different medical approach. Worse is that you must deal with the conflicting conclusions of medical research and the disagreements among the doctors themselves as to the best treatment. At first, you assume the denizens of the medical world to be infallible. You *want* them to be infallible, to say to you, "Take this remedy and you will get better." That expectation is the real dilemma of doctors;

your dilemma is that they cannot meet that expectation. They are not infallible.

Nicole Bruinsma is a doctor. She says with anguish, "Doctors have to deal with this all the time. We tell patients to take a drug that a year later researchers tell us is no good. We can only go on our best and most current information—and gut instinct." Nicole Bruinsma also had breast cancer. As a patient, a thirty-seven-year-old mother of three daughters, she had to trust her doctor's advice; as a doctor, she knew that the foundation of knowledge upon which that advice is based could shift at any moment. "That's the history of medicine," she says. "That's the way it has always been."

Doctors know that. Researchers know that. Until recently, most patients did not know that. They do now. With the information age has come direct access to medical journals, clinical studies, conference papers, theses, and books. It is ironic that the tidal wave of medical information available to everyone has exposed the fissures in actual medical knowledge.

So you now have cancer raging in your body and confusion raging in your head. You perhaps see a surgeon who recommends that the tumor be removed as soon as possible. Or maybe the recommendation is to leave the tumor in place and have radiation. Or both. Your oncologist might then advise a six-month course of chemotherapy. Or not. These doctors might say, "Do this or this, because all the studies indicate that this is the most successful procedure for your type and stage of cancer." Or you might be offered a choice: "Here are the options. Let me know what you choose."

There are now decision kits on the market to help you (and your doctor) make treatment choices. For example, in the case of breast cancer, there is a kit to help you decide whether to have a lumpectomy (removal of the tumor and surrounding tissue) or a mastectomy (removal of the whole breast). The kits are designed, says Annette M. O'Connor, professor of nursing at the University of Ottawa, for instances when "doctors need to exercise judgment and patients need to establish preference." The developers of the decision kit say that its use improves comprehension of the issue from 54 percent to 75 percent, creates more realistic expectations (28 percent to 54 percent), but doesn't really improve clarity of choice. So even with a decision kit, how on earth do you make such a decision?

Possibly, you might be given no option at all; your doctor might say, "Don't you fret about it. That's my job, I'll tell you what's best," with a metaphorical pat on the head. Or you may have to face the final non-option: "I'm sorry, we can do nothing for you. Go home and put your affairs in order."

While you are struggling with the diagnosis and the treatment choices recommended by your mainstream medical team, you are hearing about the alternative world of cancer therapies. Would this be a better route? Could you do both? More decisions. About now you realize that there seems to be a war going on, not the famous war against cancer announced by then U.S. President Nixon in 1971, but another—the Gulf War between conventional and non-conventional cancer therapies.

The medical establishment has arrogated to itself the term "conventional" to indicate accepted, proven approaches to cancer treatment. These are the mainstream therapies—surgery, chemotherapy, and radiation—which hold sway at present. "Conventional" suggests tried and true. "Tried" certainly. "True," in that they work? Not so certain. Many would say they rule the cancer-treatment stage at present not because they are so successful but because there is nothing else out there yet. Some new approaches, with the help of a huge concentration of research and investment, are struggling to hit the big time—biological (immunology) therapies, anti-angiogenesis drugs, and gene therapy, for example. They are still in the wings, though, not yet having made the leap from research through trials to practice. A few forms of immunology therapies, including some vaccines, float on the fringe of the conventional realm, but many practitioners and researchers feel they have no right to be there.

All other approaches to cancer treatment (their numbers are legion), fall into the category of "alternative or non-conventional" by virtue of two criteria: they are not one of the big three and they are not supported by the medical establishment in any formal way. These underdogs labour under various sobriquets, ranging through "complementary" (the kindest) and "unproven," to "fraudulent" and "quackery."

It is much easier to categorize mainstream cancer therapies because they fall neatly into the three approaches of surgical, drug, or radiation techniques, which pretty well define the current conventional approaches. It is not so easy to categorize alternative cancer therapies because they are so numerous. They include the "soft" ones: herbal, Chinese, vitamin, metabolic, homeopathic, electromagnetic, orthomolecular, naturopathic, nutritional, and mind/body; and the "hard" ones: experimental vaccines, immunology sera, and anti-angiogenesis drugs. Although they represent a wide range of theories and approaches, most are based on the philosophy of supporting the body in fighting the cancer, rather than mounting a direct attack.

In his TV series, *Magic or Medicine* (and his book by the same name), Toronto oncologist Dr. Robert Buckman bridges the gulf between the two worlds. A self-described conventional doctor, he puts aside training and turf to look at many other forms of medicine. With a blithe disregard for the battle lines, he slots all healing techniques into five categories. Healers can give the patient something to eat or drink; invade the body through surgery or injection of drugs; manipulate the outside of the body or apply something like a poultice; use a remote source of energy or force; or alter the patient's mind or belief. Simple as that. However, in cancer therapy, a battle line runs right through the middle of these approaches, pitching the invasive techniques against the non-invasive, the "evidence-based" techniques against the ones accepted on faith and anecdotal evidence.

And there you are, sitting on that battle front, dealing not only with your newly diagnosed cancer but with a medical war zone further complicated by the hostilities within the ranks of each of these approaches; the political battles raging over health-care costs and cuts; the fights over research money; the covert hostilities of the cancer drug industry—the list goes on. And make no mistake, you are now in the lists.

Although the three current orthodoxies of conventional cancer treatment are linked in their establishment supremacy, it was not always so. Until the sixteenth century, surgeons were barbers who cut flesh as well as hair; the real doctors were the thinkers, the professors of medicine; the surgeons were the craftsmen, nothing more. It was a development in military weapons that hastened the surgeons' climb up the medical social scale: "It was not until the Italian Wars of the sixteenth century that artillery was put to its first major sustained test, as well as its first major confrontation with the healing powers of medical science. In this contest, the long-robed contemplative professors of medicine proved unequal to the challenge. In the end, it was the humble, uneducated barber-surgeon Ambroise Paré who understood what was needed, and provided a solution. . . . It was in their perception of what constituted 'fit medicine' that the doctors of the sixteenth century made their greatest error in wound treatment. The error was due to their mistaken belief that gunshot wounds are somehow poisoned by the gunpowder, and must therefore undergo a cleansing with boiling oil" (Nuland 1995, pp. 98–99).

As so often happens in the history of medicine, an important discovery was made quite by accident. Thank God for such accidents. At the siege of Turin in 1537, Paré worked feverishly among the wounded soldiers, using the orthodox treatment of cauterizing their wounds with boiling oil. Luckily for some soldiers that night, and for future patients, he ran out of oil and instead used a "bland soothing lotion" on their smashed bodies. Eureka! Boiling oil was no longer the treatment of choice for healing wounds. With this discovery, Paré vaulted barber-surgeons onto the first rung of the ladder to their highest prominence in the 1920s and 1930s, when surgery was seen to be the answer to all medical ills. The pendulum had swung with a vengeance. One surgeon, William Arbuthnot Lane, wielded the scalpel with the same alacrity as a carpenter his saw. He advocated the removal of lengths of intestine as a solution to constipation or even as a prophylactic against "autointoxication"—"the self-poisoning which he supposed resulted from the artificialities of modern civilization" (Porter 1997a, p. 599).

The knife became the solution to almost any medical problem, but it met its match in cancer. Sigmund Freud had twenty-five operations on cancerous tissue in his mouth before succumbing to the disease in 1939. Surgical removal of cancerous organs did not stem the spread of cancer. Studies as early as 1937 indicated the same level of survival among women with breast cancer who had had a full Halsted mastectomy (removal of the breast, surrounding muscles, and portion of the chest wall) and those who had simply had the tumor removed (lumpectomy versus mastectomy, a debate that continues to this day). The apogee of heroic surgery in cancer treatment may have been an operation in 1955 when one poor fellow had both legs and his pelvis amputated in an unsuccessful effort to arrest the disease. It didn't.

Radiologists hit the medical ground running, in some instances hotly pursued by surgeons. Radiotherapy had long been popular in Europe where surgeons were not so powerful as in the United States (Patterson 1987, p. 192). Although a Canadian, John Cunningham McLennan, was knighted in 1935 for his pioneering work on radium as a treatment for cancer, it was the U.S. National Cancer Institute's growing interest, along with the huge power of the industrial-military complex, that propelled radiation cancer therapy onto center stage. It seemed to mushroom out of the collective guilt of the atomic era, proof that something good could come from such a destructive force. The dark side—culminating in the bombing of Hiroshima and Nagasaki—was counterbalanced by a wave of enthusiasm for its medical possibilities. In 1947, CBS ran a cheerful documentary, "The Sunny Side of the Atom," that dwelt on the possible medical wonders to be born out of bomb research. That same year, the American Medical Association's magazine *Hygeia* claimed that "medically applied atomic science has already saved more lives than were lost in the explosions at Hiroshima and Nagasaki" (ibid., p. 193).

Although there were some naysayers, their cautionary words were blown away in the storm of enthusiasm for technological solutions to everything. We won the war against Japan, why not against cancer? Critics, even within the National Cancer Institute (NCI) and the American Cancer Society (ACS), expressed quiet reservations that radiation therapy was at best an inexact science, at worst, highly dangerous to patients. Fifty years later, this observation still applies.

The "golden era" of chemotherapy was also born of military parentage, another explosion, not atomic but chemical, and at about the same time. In December 1943, an Allied ship carrying mustard gas blew up. Autopsies performed on the sailors who had died of the toxic effects of the liquefied gas revealed that the gas had destroyed the bone marrow and inhibited reproduction of red and white blood cells and platelets. This led to speculation that the chemical might be effective in killing other fast-growing cells such as cancer cells. A derivative of mustard gas, mustine, was the first chemotherapy drug to be developed and showed "occasional dramatic success in the treatment of what had been previously regarded as hopeless cases" (Buckman 1996, p. 296). Hodgkin's disease, even in its advanced stages, was sometimes responding to the drug.

After the war, the chief medical officer of the American Army's Chemical Warfare Division, Cornelius ("Dusty") Rhoads, went to the Sloan-Kettering Institute for Cancer Research, part of the Memorial Hospital in New York and, at the time, the biggest private cancer research facility in the world. Lewis Strauss, head of the Atomic Energy Commission in the United States in the 1940s, became a trustee of the Sloan-Kettering Institute, strengthening the medical–military connection that weaves through the history of both chemotherapy and radiation, informing attitudes and even the semantics of cancer therapy to this day. Cancer is the "enemy," against which the government has "declared war." It will be defeated with an "arsenal of weaponry," including chemical and atomic warfare. Unfortunately, the battleground for this war is not the boot of Italy or the deserts of Africa but the interior landscape of the human body.

Both Rhoads and Strauss were voluble proponents of the "agents orange" of cancer warfare during the late 1940s and 1950s, both downplaying the possible risks and dangers inherent in these approaches. Rhoads claimed that, with drug and radiation therapy, "it is no longer a question *if* cancer will be controlled, but *when* and *how soon*" (Patterson 1987, p. 196). Fifty years later it seems that it *is* a question of "if," especially if we keep trying to beat the disease with the same old weapons.

Those same old weapons, plus surgery, still hold the cancer treatment fort, to continue the military metaphor. And now you are part of that metaphor. Gentlemen/women, choose your weapons. But how? What do you base your choice on, a choice that, in your newly diagnosed state, will apparently determine whether you live forever or die by the end of the month.

This is what you hear and read about the three main cancer treatments, the information upon which you must base your decisions, your life.

Surgery

This is the best cure for in-situ cancers (cancers that have not spread), excising or "de-bulking" tumors and preventing metastases. "This therapy has been used . . . for probably 2,000 years—and to date it still offers the best chance of cure when the cancer can be totally contained in the area that is removed and has a low tendency to spread elsewhere" (Buckman 1996, p. 295).

On the other hand, it is invasive, disfiguring, often unnecessary, and rarely gets all the cancer despite the frequent claim by the surgeon that "we got it all"; according to some, surgery actually encourages the proliferation of cancer cells. When a large tumor is cut out, a scattering of small tumors spring up, nourished by blood vessels strengthened by the removal of the host tumor (sort of like cutting back a rose bush to stimulate new growth). "A microscopic miscue or careless manipulation of tumor tissue by the surgeon can 'spill' literally millions of cancer cells into the blood stream. . . . Surgery weakens immunity, places great systemic stress on the patient, and can cause sudden death" (Walters 1993, p. 14).

Chemotherapy

This is the cornerstone of modern cancer therapy. Its dramatic successes are related to Hodgkin's disease (a cancer of the lymphocytes), childhood leukemias, testicular cancer, and some forms of rare cancers. New drugs are constantly being tested for other cancers. It is the only real treatment we've got against most cancers because it can kill cancer cells already in the body systems. New important classes of chemotherapeutic drugs are on the horizon, novel drug combinations are showing promise, and progress is being made with "smart bombs"—monoclonal antibodies that target specific cancer cells as well as deliver chemotherapy and radiation directly to those cells.

On the other hand, it kills more patients than it cures, is useless for many cancers, causes secondary cancers, and is so toxic it destroys the immune system, leaving the body susceptible to other diseases, including new cancers. "To find a chemical that will make cancer disappear and leave normal tissues unharmed would be like finding a drug that you can take by mouth that will make one ear disappear and not the other" (Patterson 1987, p. 197).

Radiation

Techniques have improved dramatically over the last few years. Radiation is effective, with fewer side effects than chemotherapy (in the treatment of breast cancer, radiologists like to compare its effects with "at worst, a bad sunburn"), very powerful on the eradication of certain cancers, and is useful as a palliative measure for relief of pain in advanced cancers.

On the other hand, even in low doses, it can cause cancer and is highly invasive, painful, and disfiguring. It can only be successful in curing cancer in dosages so high as to kill the patient. It damages body organs and tissues and actually increases death rates when used as adjuvant treatment for such diseases as breast cancer.

In his elegant history of medicine, *The Greatest Benefit to Mankind*, Roy Porter sums it up: "At no time this century could a sober analyst think the cancer war was being won with the routine weaponry in the arsenal: surgery, chemotherapy and radiation" (1997a, p. 578).

The situation is much the same for alternative cancer therapies. Totally opposing claims ping-pong through the literature. Although these therapies cover a much broader spectrum of approaches than do the three major conventional treatments, their detractors usually lump them all together in one rattle-bag, claiming that, at best, they are costly, and a waste of time; at worst, they are fraudulent, futile, and fatal. Same goes for the practitioners of alternative therapies: at best, they are self-deluded; at worst, they are criminals, quacks, and murderers.

The defenders of alternative cancer therapies are usually more specific in their claims of efficacy for one or another approach. But a general theme runs through their arguments: alternative therapies usually treat the patient, not just the disease, and are far less invasive than conventional approaches. Few alternative approaches have undergone the rigors of random double-blind clinical trials. (These are studies in which patients who fit a specific set of criteria are divided into groups, each receiving a different treatment. In some trials— although rarely those testing cancer therapies—one group receives a placebo, one group is given the current "best practices" therapy, and a third receives the treatment being tested. "Double-blind" indicates that neither the patient nor the administrating doctor or nurse knows who is getting what.)

Critics of alternative therapies cite lack of scientific evidence that the therapy works. Proponents claim that the proof is empirical, based on observation of the numbers of cancer patients, many of whom have "failed" conventional methods, who do well, against all statistical odds, on non-conventional treatment.

For many people, the anguished struggle to sort out treatment options comes down to a decision whether to go with the heart or the mind. But it is not as simple as that. The debate is far too complicated to allow for a simple either/or solution. One of the murkiest areas of the debate is statistics, the be-all and end-all of science-based medicine. Beyond lies and damned lies, statistics occupy a place all their own. They are, without question, the most potent of tools. They are both the means to an end, and an end in themselves. They provide the direction for medical science, the pebbles of certainty for researchers, the handholds for doctors stranded on the ever-shifting cliff of cancer treatments. They provide the arsenal for supporting some treatments and shooting down others. But it seems that they can skewer or support just about any theory or approach, depending on who is wielding them. They can be manipulated, analyzed, shifted, and sorted to say just about anything anyone wants them to say.

From the inside of a cancer diagnosis it is hard to hang onto the one main truth about statistics: they have nothing to do with you when you become one. They apply to groups, and you are not a group. You are one. Statistics are averages, percentages, summaries, and numbers; they are mathematics, an inhuman language that bears no relevance to the reality of the individual. To translate a statistical prognosis of survival into the prognosis of an individual cancer patient is about as accurate as the famous translation of the adage "Out of sight, out of mind," which became "Invisible lunatic."

Statistics are the linguistic coinage that ensures deep misunderstanding between doctor and patient. Time and again, a cancer patient will say, "My doctor gave me six months to live (or eleven months, or three years)." Some doctors might indeed say just that. More likely, though, the doctor has said, "With your type and stage of cancer, the statistical prognosis is six months (or eleven months or three years)." There is a world of difference between these two statements, a world of difference between what the doctor says and what the patient hears. Statistics might be the actuarial shield with which doctors can protect themselves from the pain of the individual sitting before them. Unfortunately, they are also the language that increases that suffering. Statistics have no place in the consulting room.

So there you are: a cancer diagnosis has hurled you into data hell where you can find "proof" that every treatment, medical procedure, diet, exercise regimen, and therapy works. And does not work. The stats are the shrapnel that punctures hope. Beneath the strident voices of the protagonists, all persuading you that the only way is their way, you might just hear the tiny murmur of the patients who whisper, "Hey, what about us?" That murmur is growing louder as the ranks of cancer sufferers swell. "What about us? Not just our cancer, our tumors, but *us*?" Well, "us" just want our health back.

Swamped with information, claims, and counter-claims, fearful of choosing the "wrong" treatment or listening to the wrong doctor, you might begin to question whether the right to freedom of choice is worth it. It is. Ultimately, it must be your call because it is your body and your mind that are in danger of becoming the casualties, not of cancer, but of the cancer wars. So what to do? How to choose? The pat answers are, "Find a doctor you can trust. Find a treatment that puts you first and your disease second. Find a treatment that you can believe in, and believe hard. And never give up hope." Easy to say. But this is what so many cancer patients are doing. Not content to accept without demur, they seek, question, and choose.

When Anatole Broyard, literary critic and columnist for the *New York Review of Books*, was diagnosed with prostate cancer in 1989, he wrote, "When you learn that your life is threatened, you can turn toward this knowledge or away from it. I turned toward it." So have the people whose stories are told here. They have searched for the hypothetical doctor Broyard describes rather wistfully: "Just as he orders blood tests and bone scans of my body, I'd like my doctor to scan *me*, to grope for my spirit as well as my prostate. Without some such recognition, I am nothing but my illness" (Broyard 1992, p. 45). The people on these pages have searched for the treatment that will not necessarily cure their cancer, but that will at least leave them intact—a person, not a disease.

2

Do No Harm?

Your cancer journey actually starts long before the diagnosis, but often you don't know you've left home yet. You find a lump, you can't get rid of a cough, a cut won't heal. Or maybe what you thought was indigestion persists no matter what you eat or don't eat. A wisp of unease sends you to your GP. One of two things happens at this point. Your doctor either takes your symptoms seriously and refers you to a specialist and/or sends you for tests; or tells you not to worry and sends you home.

Unfortunately, despite the huge emphasis on the importance of early detection, sometimes cancers are missed and patients dismissed. Myths and misinformation can still cloak the stealthy birth of a cancer. A 1995 study of physicians and breast cancer patients across Canada found that women were often blocked from proper treatment by the inadequate knowledge and outdated attitudes of their GPs. "They are the gatekeepers to the system," noted one of the study's researchers.

"They wield enormous power. Women told us over and over of doctors, usually men, usually older, who perpetuated the myths: 'You're too young to get breast cancer' or 'Large breasts are prone to benign lumps' or 'If the lump hurts, it's not malignant.'" Wrong on all counts. You are never too young to get breast cancer. A Canadian organization, Willow Breast Cancer Support and Resource Service, has helped women as young as fourteen with the disease. Malignant tumors can develop in a breast whatever the size; and pain certainly does not equal "benign." These comfort statements often only delay the diagnosis, not negate it.

Let's say, though, that you are lucky and your doctor listens, does a thorough examination, and sends you for tests. These could be either imaging tests or blood and tissue tests. The most common imaging techniques include X-rays, CT scans (computerized tomography—really just a high-tech X-ray), MRIs (magnetic resonance imaging), nuclear medicine scans (in which a radioactive dye is injected or ingested by the patient), ultrasound (high-frequency sound waves are bounced off the target), and endoscopies (long light tubes, which function like a telescope, are inserted into the relevant body orifice).

Except for blood-related cancers such as leukemia, diagnostic blood tests do not look for cancer cells per se but for a chemical by-product of the cancer. Probably the most common test in use at the moment is the one used to determine the presence of prostate cancer, called PSA (prostate-specific antigen). A cancerous prostate produces higher quantities of PSA than a normal one; abnormally high amounts of PSA are detectable in a blood sample.

Biopsies, which are the ultimate diagnostic test for the presence of cancer cells, involve various forms of extraction of tissue for examination. A Pap smear for cervical cancer is a form of biopsy in that it consists of a scraping of cells from the cervix. An incisional biopsy takes a sample of a tumor; an excisional biopsy cuts out the whole thing; a needle biopsy aspirates tissue or fluid from a suspicious lump; and a core biopsy uses a needle with a larger core which draws more representative tissue from the lump.

A pathologist studies the sample tissue to establish if the cells are malignant, if the tumor is a primary (the originating cancer site) or secondary (a new cancer caused by cells that have spread—metastasized—to another site from the primary cancer), how abnormal the cells are, how aggressive, and how advanced. The TNM system (*T*umor size and spread, lymph *N*ode involvement, distant *M*etastases) provides the information needed for the grading and staging of the cancer, which in turn dictates the treatment of choice.

Variations and refinements of this approach continue to evolve, but these basic steps cover activities that can take several months or be fast-tracked into a matter of days. Whatever the speed, the person undergoing the tests is on a roller coaster of emotion, alternating between the highs of hope and the lows of despair and certainty that the tests are going to confirm the worst.

If they do, surgery, radiation, and chemotherapy will probably be the main offerings. Radiology and oncology specialists Brenner and Hall are admirably honest in their choice of words: "[These] are by no means the only treatment options available, but they are by far the most common, and the most tested" (1996, p. 29). They do not say "most successful" or "proven" but most "common" and "tested." As always, the semantics are crucial: "tested" is not a synonym for "proven."

Now you know you have the disease. And now you are finding out that your treatment choice, along with your odds of survival, is a crap shoot.

Carving out the Cancer

When Steve Gibbons took the appointment that his wife couldn't go to, he had a colonoscopy—not because he had any symptoms but as a precaution because of his age. He was sixty-three and healthy as a trout. He thought.

"Five feet of cable with a camera on the end. Up the butt. Within five minutes they found a tumor. Since I was already in the hospital the surgeon said, 'I can operate tomorrow.' When I came out of the anaesthetic, the surgeon was sitting on my bed, exuberant. 'I got it all,' he said. But what did he know?"

The CT scan told a different story. "The surgeon came into my room, hanging his head, embarrassed. He said, 'I'm sorry, you have tumors on the liver. Now you need chemo. That's where we pump poison into you.'"

A friend told Steve that you had to "interview" more than one doctor before making a decision on treatment. A new concept to him. "My wife's hairdresser recommended the first one. He'd been Harry Helmsley's oncologist. His opinion: 'Go for surgery—resection of the liver.'"

Steve talked to two other doctors: "They both said forget surgery, go for chemo."

Then he went to another surgeon at Sloan-Kettering who said that he was a perfect candidate for surgery. "He said, 'Without it and only with chemo, you'll live at best eighteen to twenty months.'"

"What to choose? This was my life, not a menu."

He opted for more surgery. "They opened me up and found six more small tumors undetected in the MRI. Closed me up without doing anything."

Surgery just wasn't going to cut it. He had to go back to the menu and choose again.

Surgery has been a treatment for cancer as long as there has been cancer, which is as long as recorded time. References to the disease are found in ancient Egyptian papyri, and evidence of cancer has been found in Egyptian mummies. Hippocrates, who lived in 500 B.C., is credited with naming it, "likening the long, distended veins radiating from lumps in the breast to crabs—*karkinoma* in Greek, *cancer* in Latin" (Patterson 1987, p. 12). Not only did it look like a crab, it acted like a crab: voracious, stealthy, and relentless. Hippocrates bowed to this adversary, counseling against heroic therapy. "It is better," he advised, "not to apply any treatment in cases of occult [hidden] cancer; for if treated, the patients die quickly; but if not treated, they hold out for a long time" (ibid., p. 12). There are many today who would still agree with that counsel.

Even so, surgery was used to try and stem the crab, including amputations of the female breast, but it was recognized from the beginning that cancer can travel fast, scuttling through the body looking for new sites on which to feed, and usually the scalpel is too late. In fact, it was believed that some surgeries even hastened the spread of the disease, yet another conclusion that is regaining credence. Celsus, a Roman doctor of the first century A.D., concluded, "only the beginning of a cancer admits a cure; but when 'tis settled and confirmed, 'tis incurable. . . ." (ibid., p. 12). Words as apt today as 2,000 years ago.

But surgery was pretty much the only game in town until the advent first of the therapeutic use of X-rays or radium in the early years of this century and later of chemotherapy after World War II. In 1913, Samuel Hopkins Adams wrote that the only cure for cancer was the knife, and that only if the disease was detected in its earliest stages (ibid., p. 66). But Celsus appears to have been right again. Although surgery is usually successful only if the cancer has not spread, it is still a front-line therapy for metastatic cancer.

In 1939, Sigmund Freud died in excruciating pain, following twenty-five operations for his cancer. In the summer of 1998, three bakers in Ottawa, all of whom have mouth cancer, perhaps caused by breathing the dust from the chlorinated flours of their profession, are so far facing their third round of surgery. The initial surgeries for these men were in 1993 and 1994 when they were diagnosed; at that time they each had external beam and implant radiation treatments as well as the surgical "commando procedures," as they are sometimes called, a term indicating the severity of their intent. Within twelve months, all three were suffering from radiation-induced cancers and all three had more surgery. These men now cannot breathe on their own. They speak with difficulty, their cancer continues unabated, and they are facing more surgery and a bleak prognosis. In such cases, one researcher says, "bleak prognosis" means "death. A painful, difficult death." Like Freud's, almost sixty years ago.

Burning out the Cancer

Helene Greenstein was diagnosed in 1987 with breast cancer. Mammography found the lump in her right breast: "It looked like a little throw rug: rectangular with tassels on either end," Helene says. "I also felt a lump in my left breast but the surgeon said don't worry about it. That one didn't show up in the mammogram.

"My first operation was on April 8: lumpectomy, [lymph] nodes clear" (meaning that the cancer had not spread beyond the original site). When she went to schedule her radiation treatments, she mentioned the other lump again. "After checking, they said 'Well, no, you don't have one lump in your left breast. You have two.'" Less than a week later, Helene had a second lumpectomy; this time cancer was found in one lymph node.

She was told by her doctors that now she needed chemo-therapy as well as radiation. "I had a friend who was a bio-chemist who knew of Dr. Burton's work [Dr. Burton was founder of the Immuno-Augmentative Therapy (IAT) Clinic, Bahamas]. My friend said, 'Do the IAT thing first. If it doesn't work then have chemo and radiation.' Sort of the last resort in reverse. It was good advice because I've heard that, with a ductal carcinoma, statistics say that it will come back in twenty-one years. With radiation treatment it will come back in ten. If I had had radiation, would it be back? Who knows, but I'd rather have a chance at that twenty-one-year mark."

Berris Pantaluk also has breast cancer. She was diagnosed in November 1991 at age forty-eight. With eight nodes positive, she needed chemotherapy and radiation. Berris quotes her oncologist: "You've got breast cancer. I give you a very poor prognosis. Even with chemo and radiation, you have only a 30 percent chance for recovery. I'll take you to the nurse." Berris didn't go to the nurse. She went to the Bahamas instead. For three years she took the IAT serum injections. "In February 1996, the doctor at home found another lump in my left breast. The surgeon said, 'You have five days to decide what to do: another lumpectomy with radiation or a full mastectomy with chemotherapy. Let me know.'

"I called Dr. Clement [medical consultant at the IAT Clinic] and he said, you really don't have a choice now, Berris, you must have that breast off.' So I did. And as soon as I was well enough I went back to IAT."

She had her medical records with her which indicated that the margins had not been clear—there were cancer cells beyond the tumor. "They didn't tell me that at home. Dr. Clement told me that I really did need radiation treatments. To go back home, and when my wound had healed to start the treatments. Then the immunology would have a chance." A chance to control the cancer, to keep it at bay, not a chance for a cure.

X-rays as therapeutic agents were first used in the treatment of cancer in the early years of this century, especially for surface skin cancers. The discoverer of X-rays, Wilhelm Konrad Röntgen, a physics professor at Würzburg in 1895, named them "X" because they were an unknown quantity. Their long-term effects unfortunately remained unknown for decades. X-rays were still casually used in the 1950s to measure children's feet when buying shoes. I remember well the September, new-school-year ritual—new pencils, new books, and new shoes. At the shoe store in our small town—and no doubt in small and large towns all over Canada and the United States—the highlight was sliding your bare feet into the slot at the bottom of a large machine. When the salesman flicked a switch, you peered down the viewer to see the bones in your feet light up, green skeletons glowing with radioactivity.

An X-ray cure for a cancer patient was reported as early as 1899, but "it soon became clear that the rays themselves caused cancer" (Patterson 1987, p. 64).

The use of radium seemed more promising. Discovered almost at the same time as X-rays in 1898 by Marie Curie and her husband, Pierre, radium provoked great interest among physicians as the basis for a miracle cure for cancer. However, it was not to be. In fact, "Therapeutic enthusiasm outran caution, and the dangers of radiotherapy were determined at great cost to patients and radiographers alike" (Porter 1997a, p. 608). Many died from exposure to radioactivity.

With the advent of radiotherapies came more turf wars. The proponents of these new approaches to cancer treatment found themselves nose to nose with physicians and surgeons who decried the approach, claiming that "this vogue for radium encouraged a new wave of quackery and stopped patients from undergoing necessary surgery" (Patterson 1987, p. 66). They were up against some tenacious defenders though.

One researcher insisted that radium could "extend life, restore vigor of youth, prevent wrinkles, produce new hair on bald heads, and possibly a third set of natural teeth" (*Chicago Tribune*, December 1922, as quoted in ibid., p. 66).

The major developments in radiology treatment since the 1930s have been in the technology—more sophisticated machines, computers that allow more accurate targeting of the cancer site and more precise calibration of dosages, and different methods of delivering the treatment through implants.

In current cancer treatment, radiation therapy is often used as adjuvant therapy to surgery, a kind of mopping-up exercise. The rationale is that radiation will kill any malignant cells left over after a tumor has been removed, either at the tumor site itself or in the adjacent lymph nodes, thus reducing the possibility of recurrence and improving survival. As one commentator remarks: "Nice hypothesis, shame about the facts." In July 1998, the British medical journal *Lancet* published the results of a meta-analysis indicating that radiation treatment for lung cancer patients, a common practice, actually does harm rather than good. An international team of researchers combined information gathered from nine studies over the last thirty years (involving 2,128 lung cancer patients) and found that patients who had been radiated after surgery were 21 percent more likely to die within two years than those who had surgery only. The detrimental effect was worse in patients in the early stages of the disease (Stewart 1998, p. 1).

Radiation has been particularly lauded in the treatment of childhood cancers. Its success comes not without cost. "In summary, although long-term survival has been achieved in a number of children [through radiotherapy] who are now entering adulthood, many of these individuals have major endocrinopathies" (Green and D'Angio 1992, p. 61). "The deleterious skeletal effects of radiation can be minimized by adopting certain routines. . . ." (ibid., p. 69). "Radiation injury to the eye in children treated for retinoblastoma, rhabdomyosarcoma, and other malignant orbital tumors is usually severe and visually significant" (ibid., p. 19). Green and D'Angio issue a heartfelt plea: "Vigilance is essential if the blossoms of success in pediatric oncology are not to bear bitter fruit. Cure is not enough" (ibid., p. 5).

Evidence of radiation-caused cancers continues to cloud the issue of radiation as cancer treatment, a cruel irony that fuels the debate on its efficacy and the ethics of using it in treatments of some cancers for short-term gain versus long-term pain. "Usually radiation induced cancer does not turn up for 20 years," say Brenner and Hall, adding defensively, "We certainly know more about the risks of radiation-induced cancer than we do about the risks of cancer from chemicals, such as chemotherapy agents. . . ." (1996, p. 13).

Poisoning the Cancer

Don Mosteller has prostate cancer. "The surgeon who operated on me said, 'We got it all,'" Don says. "I guess they all say that, because now it has spread to my liver, lungs, and hip bones." Four years after diagnosis, he is short of breath and coughs a lot when he speaks. His voice is weakening. It's reedy, like an old man's voice. Don is in his forties.

"I heard about this place [the IAT Clinic] a year ago. I should have come then. But I was feeling OK. Suddenly, though, I started to lose weight; the cancer was having a field day. It was frightening. I turned around one day and I was barely there."

His doctor back home in Indiana wanted him to take chemotherapy. He told Don it would give him a 25 percent chance to live eleven more months, but the side effects would be horrendous—hair loss, vomiting, fatigue, weakness, joint pain, organ damage. . . .

"This is living?" Don whispers. "Without chemo, they gave me a one percent chance of survival for the same period. But with chemo you open yourself to a Pandora's box of ills."

"The doctor told him, 'Without chemo you will die quite soon. Go home and do what you have left to do,'" his wife Kathy, says, her mouth twisting in pain.

Don seriously considered taking chemotherapy. He was within three days of starting the treatment when a sentence in a book he was reading jumped off the page at him. "The author, who had had cancer, wrote that whatever treatment you take it shouldn't do you harm. You should try and work with your body, not against it," Don says. He stops again, fighting for breath. The pauses that punctuate his speech add impact to his words, chosen carefully to husband his strength. "That . . . about . . . rules . . . out . . . chemo."

In 1991, Joanne Ely found a lump on her chest; her family doctor said it was fatty tissue and not to worry about it. She noticed it changing and went back to the doctor, who was rather testy, she felt: "He said, 'No it hasn't changed, you don't know what you are talking about, there's nothing to worry about.'"

Joanne worried. At her husband's urging, she went to another doctor, and her week went like this: Monday: doctor's appointment: "You're right—that lump has to come out, fast." Thursday: surgery to remove lump. Friday: diagnosis—carcinoma of the chest wall.

Joanne was told that the lump was malignant and more

surgery was required. One week later she went back into hospital for five days of chemotherapy followed by radiation.

"I was OK for a while," says Joanne, "but I was mad that my doctor didn't believe me, didn't move faster at the beginning of all this."

Three and a half years later, a persistent cough announced recurrence—the cancer had spread into her lung and lymph system. This time the chemotherapy treatments put her into hospital for twenty-three days. "I nearly died from the treatment," Joanne says. "But it didn't stop that cough."

It was at this point that Joanne's battle became more than just a fight against cancer; she found herself in the no man's land of conflicting medical advice, where the casualties are not cancer cells but trust in the experts. She and her husband went to Johns Hopkins for a second opinion on what to do about the metastases in her lung. There she was told that she had had her absolute limit of Adriamycin, described guilelessly by one doctor as a chemotherapeutic drug that sometimes works "when gentler drugs are no longer effective."

Back home, her oncologist recommended what he called an "experimental" regimen. One of the drugs would be Adriamycin. "I said, 'Wait a minute, at Johns Hopkins I was told I couldn't have that and you're wanting to give it to me?' And his response? 'Uh-oh!' Like a kid who's been caught out doing something he shouldn't. That's all? 'Uh-oh'? He didn't recommend it again."

Adriamycin (the proprietary name for doxorubicin) is commonly used in treatment of a range of cancers; its side effects include all the usual ones—nausea, vomiting, hair loss—plus damage to the heart. As the cumulative effect increases, so does the risk of congestive heart failure (Moss 1995, p. 182). There is "accumulating evidence of late cardiotoxicity in patients treated with Adriamycin. Children and young adults who appear to be perfectly well nonetheless show signs of cardiac dysfunctions. . . . Instances of sudden cardiac failure in women at the time of parturition are becoming more than the occasional anecdote" (Green and D'Angio 1992, p. 5).

Joanne says, "Later, we saw a letter in my medical file that sent me through the roof. It took me forever to get my records; they didn't want to give them to me when I said I was going to take an alternative cancer therapy. The letter was from my oncologist to one of my other doctors. It was very specific; it said, right out, that chemo would not help at this point anyway, whatever combination of drugs it was. But they gave me chemo anyway. They still went ahead and gave it to me."

In 1992, Edwina Smith was diagnosed with an aggressive form of ovarian cancer. Since then she has had a barrage of different chemotherapies which are keeping her one step ahead of the cancer. She is willing to continue with these debilitating treatments despite the nausea and pain, enduring the regular bites out of her life, as long as they pay back enough normal living to balance the months lost to treatment. At the same time, she is taking an experimental cancer vaccine which seems to be helping her immune system combat the ravages of both the cancer and the chemo.

Three patients with three different chemotherapy experiences: Don rejected it from the outset; Joanne rejected a continuation of it; and Edwina continues with chemotherapy in conjunction with an alternative therapy. They represent thousands of patients' experiences. It is no easy decision to reject a form of treatment that is so integral to mainstream cancer therapy, so enmeshed with issues other than whether it works. But the endurance of a high-dose chemotherapy regimen certainly gives new meaning to Dylan Thomas's famous line, "Do not go gentle into that good night" but perhaps go forever bald into eternity.

"Chemotherapy" means, simply, the treatment or control of disease with drugs. Technically, Aspirin is a form of chemotherapy. However, the term has come to be associated almost exclusively with cancer treatment. The word itself was coined in 1907 by the chemist Paul Ehrlich (1854–1915) who is remembered not only for developing chemotherapy, "pinning his faith on the creation of artificial antibodies" (Porter 1997a, p. 448) rather than natural substances, but also for his formulation of salvarsan 606. Developed in 1907 for intravenous use in the treatment of syphilis, the drug was acclaimed as the "new science" of drug use (Moss 1995, p. 15). Its mixed success is eerily prescient of current chemotherapies. It did appear remarkably effective, transforming syphilis treatment, but its high toxicity, its painful and prolonged administration, not to mention its arsenic base, finished off several patients. By 1914, 109 deaths had been attributed to salvarsan 606 (ibid.).

With a single phrase, Ehrlich dictated the direction of the projectile of chemotherapy research down through the twentieth century. He talked of "the magic bullet"—a hypothetical drug that would zero in on a disease with the specificity of a heat-seeking missile. Salvarsan was to be the "magic bullet" to kill off syphilis, and the search was on for another to eradicate cancer. The metaphors changed with the decades—that single bullet escalated into a full-scale armory with Nixon's declaration of war against cancer in 1971—but the vision remains at the heart of chemotherapy research and production: to find that hypothetical drug to knock out the disease while leaving the patient intact.

The golden era of chemotherapy dawned in a swirl of mustard-gas clouds sent skyward from an explosion on board a ship carrying chemical warfare materials in 1943. Despite its inauspicious genesis, the possibilities it held out for medical science appeared rosy, and its arrival on the scene as an agent not of death but of life was greeted with almost universal enthusiasm, especially among the media. The few dissenting voices were lost in the roar of the postwar celebration of the might of modern science. Faith in chemical solutions to medical problems—in most cases, well-founded—was turning western society into a drug culture, not of needles in the streets but of heady progress in the eradication of diseases that until now had stalked the earth victorious. Streptomycin was proving to be the first agent ever to have an effect on tuberculosis. Penicillin was truly a wonder drug, revolutionizing treatment of a host of diseases. In the early 1950s came the discovery of DNA, the material that controls cell division and replication. This was a truly exciting breakthrough, allowing cancer researchers to move into the whole new territory of genetics.

In such a context, surely it was now just a matter of time before a wonder drug was found to cure cancer. "Inevitably, as I see it, we can look forward to something like a penicillin for cancer, and I hope within the next decade," Rhoads declared in 1953 (Patterson 1987, p. 196). The influential Sidney Farber, a Harvard professor of pathology, lent his voice in support of chemotherapy, calling it "the greatest mobilization of resources—man, mineral, animal, and money—ever undertaken to conquer a single disease" (ibid.). His words describe the chemotherapy research complex of the 1990s as easily as that of the 1940s. Fifty years later, the "mobilization of resources" is even more gigantic, but the magic bullet still remains nothing more than a catchy metaphor.

Chemotherapy has not lived up to its press. The spin doctors, both the medical and the media versions, of those early years did chemotherapy a disservice, encouraging expectations that "it"—singular—would cure cancer—also singular.

But cancer is not one single disease, predictable in its cause, progress, and cure. It is a collection of diseases that cannot be killed by a single bullet. And chemotherapy is not a single drug but a range of chemicals. The semantics of the simplistic had set chemotherapy up for a fall.

The next decades did see some successes. About thirty drugs were tested and found useful in treatment, especially in children's cancers, leukemias, Hodgkin's disease, and histiocytic lymphomas—systemic diseases untreatable by radiation or surgery. In the broad range of cancers, these successes are a pretty meagre basis for claims that chemotherapy is the answer. Yet proponents did just that.

This belief in chemotherapy's potential continued into the early 1980s. But as the years passed and a cure for cancer did not bubble forth from the springs of chemotherapy, its critics became more vocal. These were not just the thousands of cancer patients whose disappointment in the lack of progress was sharpened by their own looming mortality. The criticisms were coming from physicians and scientists. Some objected to the huge cost of research and testing and worried about the influence of the players in the cancer industry, in particular the pharmaceutical companies whose profits increased with each patented drug; others stressed the horrific toxic effects of the drugs; still others complained that this total focus on drug therapy effectively closed out other viable approaches. The defenders of chemotherapy mostly dismissed the critics of pharmaceutical companies as paranoid, and claimed that the side effects of the drugs were a small price to pay for the end result, and opined that there *was* no other viable approach.

It is harder now to find such unambiguous proponents of chemotherapy as the be-all answer to cancer. Defenders of the faith are more cautious; qualifiers have crept into their sentences. Chemotherapy works on *some* cancers. Or they make sweeping statements that on the surface seem positive, but on closer scrutiny sound positively odd. "The good news is that chemotherapy treatment has become quite sophisticated. Many, many thousands of people receive chemotherapy today, and many find that their treatments result in fewer and milder side effects than they imagined. . . . Many people don't lose weight, and not everyone loses all his or her hair. That said, it is important to note that, like many medical treatments, chemotherapy has not attained absolute perfection" (Drum 1998, pp. 1–2). This is a defense? However, the author appears to grow more hopeful: "Everyone doesn't survive cancer. But almost everyone survives chemotherapy. . . ." (ibid., p. 10).

At a public-awareness event held by the Alberta Breast Cancer Foundation in Edmonton, a senior medical oncologist from a large cancer research centre in the United States took me gently to task when I said that we still did not have a cure for breast cancer. He said to the audience, "Despite what Ms. Williams has just told you, we *can* cure breast cancer." It turned out what he meant was, as long as it doesn't come back. The problem is with metastatic disease. With recurrence, he said, then we are not sure of a cure. This bright, personable, well-meaning research oncologist had dedicated his every waking hour to clinical studies of high-dose treatments with the drug Taxol; he was a man used to dealing with numbers, not people; doctors, not patients. He had charts and graphs and statistics. His research was "scientifically vigorous," the stamp of approval offered by his peers. He told me before the event that he had never spoken to a lay audience before, only to doctors and medical scientists. Perhaps his claim made sense to them but not to this group which included many women with breast cancer, both first time and metastatic. There was a stillness in the hall as they tried to digest this Alice in Wonderland logic. Yes, we can cure breast cancer as long as there is no recurrence. His statement, backed by the weight of science, went politely unchallenged.

In the early 1990s, Taxol was heralded as yet another breakthrough in breast cancer treatment, a drug that would cure the disease. Headlines boldly proclaimed, "Finally the good news about breast cancer." Taxol is derived from the bark of the Pacific yew tree—some would suggest that with such lineage it fits right into the alternative therapy camp. Along with Taxotere, a semi-synthetic derivative from the needle of the European yew tree, it is one of the newer breed of aggressive chemotherapies being tested in clinical trials on women with metastatic breast or ovarian cancer. Some recent studies indicate that such high-dose chemotherapy could be improving women's survival rates by 26 percent (*Toronto Star* 1998). Others indicate less positive results, suggesting that survival without recurrence is only about 4 percent higher (Bujold 1996, p. 13). The common side effects of these drugs can be horrific. For Taxotere, one medical journal lists hair loss, joint and muscle pain, skin rash, fever, fluid retention, nausea, vomiting, diarrhea, neutropenia (reduction of white blood cells), anaemia, mouth ulcers, and neurological reactions (ibid., pp. 13–14). Then there is the severest side effect of all—death.

Phase 1 clinical trials were conducted on Taxol as early as 1983, but a high incidence of "severe hypersensitivity reaction led to premature closing" of many of these trials. Perhaps not premature enough for many of the subjects.

The debilitating effects and apparent lack of real progress with surgery, radiation, and chemotherapy in cancer treatment raise the question "Why do we persevere so unswervingly in the same direction?"

First of all, some would argue that there *is* progress. For example: "Despite our incomplete understanding of why the genetic mutations occur . . . and how they result in leukemia, the disease in children is now often cured by combination chemotherapy. The conquest of childhood leukemia stands as one of the cardinal achievements of modern oncology" (Groopman 1997, p. 92).

But at what cost? Behind the proud statistics claiming success in curing childhood leukemia with chemotherapy (leukemia is the poster boy for proponents of chemotherapy treatment at the moment, being one of the few cancers that can actually be "cured" by chemotherapy) is the reality of an incredibly painful treatment often with a permanently debilitating impact on the patient's health.

Dr. Groopman, a self-described "physician-scientist," provides an unflinching description of the horrors of the treatment which "cures" an eight-year-old boy with myeloblastic leukemia:

> Matt received a tightly choreographed succession of toxic drugs, each with a different mechanism of action against the leukemia but each with deleterious effects on his normal tissues. Adriamycin: the cranberry-coloured infusion that, while shattering the DNA of the leukemic cells, removed all Matt's hair and weakened his growing heart. Ara-C: deceptively clear and transparent but responsible for ulcerating Matt's mouth and damaging his cerebellum, the balance centre of his brain, while interfering with the reproduction of the blasts. 6-TG: yet another toxic weapon against the blasts' reproductive machinery that also inflamed Matt's liver" (ibid., p. 94).

It took three intensive courses of these chemotherapies to bring the leukemic count to zero. Then the child had to go through three more intensive cycles of chemotherapy, and then six months of maintenance treatment because "[l]eukemic cells are devious and likely to hide (ibid. p. 97).

Matt's treatment lasted eighteen months, followed by three years of monitoring, blood tests, physicals, and periodic, excruciating bone-marrow exams to be sure the cancer had gone. It also took Matt those years to recover from the treatment and the residual toxicities from the high doses of chemotherapy. Five years after his initial diagnosis and three and a half years after his "cure," the child contracted HIV from one of his many blood transfusions. His immune system, so compromised by chemotherapy, had no resistance to the AIDS virus, leaving him prey to opportunistic infections. He died of meningitis at the age of thirteen. This case would go into the books as "cured" leukemia.

So the progress in "beating cancer" is not enough, and not nearly as much as we are led to believe. Here is a doctor talking of doctors: "The other day I heard on the evening news that there's been considerable progress again in cancer research. This is, I assure you, the absolute crap that you hear every few months. Cancer research has been on the brink of a Major Breakthrough for the last thirty or forty years and the funny thing is that everybody believes this without anything ever breaking through" (Keizer 1996, p. 292).

There is a desperate need to believe that we must be on the right track. If not, imagine the chaos, imagine the pain of knowing that you have urged loved ones to submit to a therapy that not only is brutal but doesn't work. Imagine the resounding crash on Wall Street when the pharmaceutical companies in the business of producing chemotherapeutics suddenly find their stocks worthless. Imagine the research facilities closing their doors because their grants are suddenly not forthcoming. Imagine the enormous changes required in teaching facilities, in hospitals, in attitudes, in insurance. It is just too big a task to turn the ship of cancer care. "Orthodox medicine is unthinkable without its research centres and teaching hospitals served by armies of paramedics, technicians, ancillary staff, managers, accountants and fund-raisers, all kept in place by rigorous professional hierarchies and codes of conduct. The medical machine has a programme dedicated to the investigation of all that is objective and measurable and to the pursuit of high-tech, closely monitored practice. It has acquired extraordinary momentum" (Porter 1997a, p. 629). The momentum appears to keep the status quo cancer treatments steaming along despite their dismal track record in many areas. An increasing number of people, including patients, practitioners, and politicians, think that that momentum, no matter how big the industry resting on it, is not a good enough reason to keep from trying to turn that ship in another direction.

Here you are, then, a well-behaved passenger, dutifully taking your chemo, your radiation, your reassurances . . . and your recurrences. Your cancer continues unabated. Or perhaps it stalls for a bit, then surges into a new part of your body. There's no harbor in sight, so you decide to jump ship, choosing a smaller and, some would say, much leakier vessel. It is a tough decision to abandon that liner with its bridge full of commanding captains, a comfort in their authoritative white uniforms, even when they argue about which direction to steer. You are sailing solo now. But like so many patients who speak from direct experience, you conclude there is no heart in this machine, and you turn away from the high-tech world of establishment cancer care, searching for answers and recovery in a world where you are recognized as a person, not a disease.

Your quest now brings you to total reliance on your own judgment and a bewildering array of options. You might rely on homeopathic or holistic remedies, including herbs and teas and tinctures. You might include vitamin therapies and detoxifying diets. You might practice Chinese medicine or Ayurveda, perhaps the oldest existing medical system, enlisting your mind in driving the cancer from your body. You might turn to acupuncture, immunology, vaccines, bioelectric therapies, oxygen therapies, or 714-X. Or you might combine alternative approaches with a conventional treatment, but keep it a secret, fearful of your doctor's scorn or refusal to continue treating you. Now you are in the world where conventional medicine, like the early mapmakers, pencils in "Here be monsters," the outposts, some physically beyond the reach of regulatory control, some figuratively beyond the bastions of orthodox cancer treatments. In the last few years, the routes to these outposts are growing busier. You meet more than the occasional traveler, searching for other ways to deal with a disease that has danced rings around us for centuries.

The Immuno-Augmentative Therapy Clinic is one of these outposts. Politically, geographically, and historically it has been isolated from the mainstream. Its story is both unique and eerily typical of cancer treatment modalities that won't toe the line.

3

Beyond the Pale: The Immuno-Augmentative Therapy Clinic, Part I

Eleanor Britton's journey to the Immuno-Augmentative Therapy Clinic in the Bahamas actually started months earlier on a flight from Malaysia to her home in Scotland. A tickly cough she'd had on and off for weeks became more persistent, aggravated, she thought, by the plane's air-filter system.

"You should see about that cough," said her husband, Bill.

Two months later Eleanor was diagnosed with lung cancer.

"How long does my wife have?" Bill asked the oncologist, who was also a good friend.

"Short end of six months."

Eleanor was given two lots of chemotherapy. "Will this work?" Bill asked.

"No," said the oncologist.

"What I didn't ask was 'Why are you giving it to her, then?'" Britton says. "I was so totally focused on finding something that might work, I didn't question, I just started to search for another way."

The Internet and word of mouth led him to the Immuno-Augmentative Therapy Clinic in Freeport. The information on the Internet was totally negative, so much so that it piqued Bill's interest. Just what was the story here? Something didn't ring true. He researched further and talked to IAT patients in the United States with the same cancer as his wife's.

Britton told the oncologist, still a friend, "We are going to the Bahamas."

The oncologist said, "Let me tell you a story about one of my patients—a true story. He had cancer, said he was going to the Andes where they could cure him. A diet of nuts and grapes or something. I told him, 'Don't you think if nuts and grapes could cure cancer, we'd do that here?' But he wouldn't listen. He sold his house, went to the Andes and died. So now instead of his wife just not having a husband, she doesn't have a home either. Don't go, Bill."

Bill: "So, what do we do?"

Oncologist: "There's no solution."

Sod that. Bill brought his wife to the Bahamas. Friends and relations all said it was a lunatic thing to do—they expected never to see her again.

In the taxi from the airport to the Princess Hotel in the Freeport International Bazaar, a maze of shops and restaurants and casinos, a featured tourist attraction of the island, Britton asked the driver, "Have you heard of this IAT Clinic?"

"Mon," the driver said, turning full around in his seat, "I's takes them there in wheelchairs and stretchers and they comes out jumpin'."

On their arrival at the clinic, Bill and Eleanor stood in the parking lot, took some pictures, hesitated about going in. The one-storey building, painted pink—the establishment color in the Bahamas—sits well back from the street behind two sets of open gates. Flowering shrubs skirt its walls; small, curtained windows sit high under the eaves. The front entrance door is smooth, solid steel.

After flying halfway around the world to get here, Bill and Eleanor found that walking through that door was the longest part of the journey, a tangible commitment to the unknown. They hadn't told anyone at the clinic they were coming. They didn't know if Eleanor would be accepted as a patient; nor did they know whether she would take IAT as her therapy. They had booked for two weeks; if they didn't like what they saw, they could at least have a bit of a holiday.

Bill describes that day with a kind of awe, even after more than a year and all that has happened since: "I asked a chap coming out of the building, 'Are you a patient here?' He said, 'Yes I am, I've been coming here eight years. Back home they said I wouldn't survive another month.' He had the grin of a Cheshire cat. 'Fooled them, didn't I?'

"And then another chap came out with his wife. Same story. Doctors back in the States had given him eight or nine months to live. He'd been playing golf the day before we met him, and he'd been living a lot longer than eight or nine months. Then another chap came up to me and said, 'You look like I looked three years ago. You don't know whether to go in or not, do you?' He took me by the arm and he said, 'I'll take you in and introduce you to the nurses.'

"I said, 'It's not me, it's my wife who has cancer.'

"'She's too pretty to have cancer, you both come with me.' And we did.

"I only needed to walk in the door and I saw a place that was not a conventional hospital. People weren't all sitting there waiting, anxious, who's next, looking down, keeping to themselves. Here everyone was talking and moving about, it was just hustle and bustle and almost chaos and I liked it."

They stayed in the Bahamas for three months.

"Eleanor was so poorly when we first got here, she couldn't walk the length of this room without becoming breathless. She was having fluid drained off—she had eight pints, then six pints, and then just before we left, four pints taken off her lungs. She'd had no surgery because the cancer was in the fluid, it was everywhere, it was outside and inside the lung. She loved the sun, and in the swimming pool, the water would support her body. At first, she would stand with one foot on the bottom and take a few strokes. By the time we left, she was swimming fifty lengths of that pool. *I* can't do fifty lengths of that pool. . . ."

Immuno-augmentative therapy is a biological treatment using cytokines obtained from the normal blood of healthy donors. Administration of these fractions is by self-subcutaneous injections, and the dosage is calculated by daily assay of the patient's blood.

The Cancer Dictionary defines biological therapy, or immunotherapy, as "the newest anticancer treatment, still primarily investigational, which uses biological response modifiers (BRMs), the body's own immune system, to fight cancer. Substances, some occurring naturally in the body and others made in the lab, are used to boost, direct, or restore normal defences of the body" (Altman and Sarg 1992, p. 26). The major BRMs are antibodies, monoclonal antibodies, vaccines, colony stimulating factors (CSFs), and cytokines. Immuno-augmentative therapy falls within the last category.

Biological cancer therapies, then, unlike chemotherapy and radiation, do not attack the cancer cells directly, but attempt to bolster the patient's immune system in order to control or destroy the cancer.

The IAT view is that while each cancer is unique to the patient who has it, what is common is a deficiency in the immune system that ordinarily would keep the cancer in check.

This does not mean that the entire immune system is weak or inadequate but that the controlling mechanism that deals specifically with cancer is lacking. Whether the cancer has been caused originally by a genetic defect, environmental factors, or whatever, this deficiency allows the cancer to grow. IAT therefore treats the competence of the immune system with the goal of restoring it to a level where it can control the disease.

Although sharing the same philosophical base of boosting the patient's immune system rather than directly attacking the cancer, immuno-augmentative therapy is not quite the same as the "mainstream" immunology therapies that are garnering attention these days.

IAT's medical consultant, Dr. John Clement, says, "We are not talking about cellular immunology here, but one step lower. Our treatment is humoral in nature—meaning it relates to solutions. We are dealing with cytokines [*cyto* is Greek for "cell"; *kineses* means "motion"], the substances produced by cells. . . . Immunology works at the cellular level . . . tagging the T cells or stem cells with certain things to enable them to reject tumors. This is at a different level. I don't know of any other work being done in humoral immunity, really."

The basis of IAT is four factors isolated from human blood: tumor antibody factor (also called tumor necrosis factor or TNF), tumor complement factor (TCF), deblocking protein factor (DPF), and blocking protein factor (BPF).

"Our biological treatment uses sera prepared from human blood," says Dr. Clement. "Tumor necrosis factor has been known for thirty years. It kills cancer cells in animals, it kills cells in cultures; we know that this stuff works, right? And it's part of the immune system in everybody. It attacks cells that shouldn't be there."

The process is similar to the body's attempt at rejecting an organ transplant. It recognizes a foreign invasion and tries to protect itself. Hence the medication people must take who have been given a new heart or kidney.

"The problem is that with some people . . . unfortunately, cancer has perfected a method of turning off the body's own rejection system so that when the body starts killing cancer cells, it perceives the cell death as something not right and puts out a protein that blocks the TNF.

"What we do is take a sample of the patient's blood and we assay TNF, which we call 'antibody' so people will understand what we're talking about. This was one of the criticisms of Burton [the founder of IAT], that he used loose terminology, but what can you say to a patient, 'We're going to give you some mouse tumor necrotising factor'?

"You can imagine the reaction—'Oh my god, don't come near me. . . .' We assay the patient's TNF and the blocking proteins that are present. The figures measuring the blockers indicate the TNF activity."

The patient is given a protein (an extraction from the blood of a healthy donor) the equivalent molecular weight of the TNF, similar enough to make the blockers think that it's the same thing. This "deblocker" knocks out the blocking protein, in a sense leveling the playing field. The serum given to the patient includes "kill factor" TNF which goes in to nail the cancer, as well as a complement to encourage a complete chemical reaction.

The balance of these four factors is arrived at through analysis of the patient's blood and a formula worked out by Lawrence Burton. He refined his work over thirty years, starting in 1955 with work on isolating naturally occurring proteins found in blood. He worked with lab mice and over the years factored in the experiences of his patients, adjusting and monitoring the formula constantly to arrive at the correct balance of the four factors to be administered to each patient.

Since IAT is an outpatient facility, patients gather each day from their temporary homes all over Freeport, rising with the sun for the early morning blood draw, a common enough medical ritual in every hospital or treatment center in the world. Patients become pincushions no matter what brand of medicine is being practiced. But at IAT, the blood map is read for different signs. Within a couple of hours the analysis of each patient's blood has provided the recipe for a customized balance of ingredients for his or her own treatment for the day. New patients stay for ten to twelve weeks. Returning patients have two or three weeks of this regimen, with an additional blood pull in the afternoons, before they return home with their supply of serum for home maintenance therapy.

By noon, the clinic is quiet, most of the patients gone. The phones ring a lot. People call from all over the world, "My son has lymphoma—can we come right away?" Or, "The doctors here say they have nothing more to give me. I have lung cancer. Can you do anything?" Or, "My wife has breast cancer. It's spread to the bones. I want to know how successful your treatment is for breast cancer. Can I talk to other IAT patients to find out how they've been doing?"

The clinic does no diagnostics itself. Patients must submit their medical records, including diagnosis, pathology reports, history of treatment to date, present medications, such as high-dose steroids and pain-control drugs, and complete blood count and blood chemistry records. With that input, Dr. Clement says, "We can give the patient an idea if we can help them. . . . I make an assessment based on particular criteria. We must have a patient who is well enough to . . . attend as an outpatient and we must have some hope that we can help them. There are certain diagnoses where we know we are not going to be able to help and then there is no point in coming. It would be fruitless for them and it would be a waste of money and a waste of time."

Patients with fast-growing cancers are not accepted at IAT because the treatment cannot get ahead of the cancer growth. About 10 percent of the patients who apply to come are turned down. For instance, Dr. Clement says, "We know that we are not going to have much time to help people with small-cell lung cancer, which has a doubling rate of thirty-three days. . . . The only hope for people with SCLC is chemotherapy, and that can buy them a bit of time but only a little bit of time."

The clinic does not accept children for treatment now. "So many of the childhood cancers—leukemia in particular, are being cured by other methods," says Dr. Clement. "There have been big breakthroughs in the treatment of children's cancers . . . and chemotherapy seems to help them. The ones who aren't helped [by chemotherapy] we can't help either."

The cost of the treatment is US$7,500 for the first month, then $700 a week for the rest of the time the patient is at the clinic, then $50 a week for the serum for home maintenance. This sounds like a hefty price tag. It *is* a hefty price tag although, IAT defenders point out, it is far less costly than conventional cancer treatment if a patient doesn't have health insurance.

The high cost of alternative cancer therapies is a criticism raised often. There is no question, alternative therapies are expensive, well beyond the means of most. But there is more than one issue here. The first is that *all* cancer treatment is expensive now, alternative and conventional. What makes conventional therapies seem less so is the presence of medical insurance, and since most alternative therapies are not recognized or approved by the medical regulatory authorities, the insurance companies won't cover them.

In the United States, medical insurance is moving rapidly toward managed care—hybrid arrangements that integrate, to different degrees, health insurance and health-care delivery. The theory is that they reduce the cost of insurance premiums and service costs. In practice, they have a virtual stranglehold on the entire medical complex, earning $952 billion a year and going "calmly about the business of eliminating one treatment after another . . ." (Glasser 1998, p. 35). The percentage of insured Americans who are enrolled with managed care groups has risen from 29 percent in 1988 to 73 percent in 1995 (United States 1999). Now, about 160.3 million people are insured through Health Management Organizations (HMOs), but coverage is restricted to medical services provided by the individual organization's group of hospitals and doctors. Patients are not allowed to seek conventional treatment, let alone alternative approaches, beyond their HMO's network of services.

Forty-eight million Americans are in private plans, most of which will not cover alternative therapies. Nor will Medicare or Medicaid.

In Canada, the major arms of cancer therapy—chemotherapy, surgery, radiation, and some experimental therapies within clinical trials—are still covered by medical insurance, either private or government but, as in the United States, not alternative therapies. With a few exceptions—for example, the Canadian alternative therapy Naessens's 714-X, if prescribed by doctors under Health Canada's Special Access Program, might be eligible for coverage—alternative therapies are a direct out-of-pocket expense to the patient.

In a straight comparison, leveling the playing field by factoring out insurance, alternative therapies are not more expensive than conventional ones; in fact, they are often far less so, a point obscured by the role played by insurance in the conventional treatment world. One patient told me that, without coverage, his six-month course of chemotherapy would have cost him $100,000 at an American hospital. Another cancer patient crashed into the harsh reality of the cost of conventional treatment without insurance when she came from the Middle East to a hospital in Texas for surgery to remove a cancer metastasis to the brain. When she and her husband arrived, with $75,000 to pay for the operation, the hospital cancelled the surgery because they were short $5,000. The husband's promise to bring the rest of the money within the next few days went unheeded. These were the rules. No money up front, no surgery.

Even so, providers of alternative therapies are singled out for their exorbitant costs. The charge is usually that they are selling the patients a bill of goods, useless therapies, and false hope. But even when empirical evidence suggests that their therapies are efficacious, they are still condemned, sometimes for charging anything at all. Commenting on my article on alternative therapies in *Homemaker's* magazine, a physician from Calgary wrote: "You might of [sic] mentioned in your article what people pay for IAT therapy. The sad fact is that if the people who advocated for these sorts of treatments were true humanitarians they would be making them available for next to nothing. . . ." I wondered if this doctor provided his services for "next to nothing." His remarks underscore the double standard often applied to alternative health practitioners. Somehow, it is acceptable that doctors in the conventional world charge fees (either directly, as is happening for an increasing number of medical services, or through insurance), but it is immoral for alternative practitioners to do the same.

IAT is not defensive about its fees. It is a private company with no government funding and no research grants. It must make money to stay in business. And until medical insurance companies are persuaded to cover its services, most patients pay directly. Some say it's a small price to pay for regaining their health, others are bitter that insurers won't consider coverage. "It would be a lot cheaper for them," one patient, an insurance agent himself, said. "Think how much money they'd save by covering IAT treatments rather than, say, a bone-marrow transplant. We're talking $20,000 instead of $150,000. And odds are, with much better results." His numbers for the cost of a bone-marrow transplant may be a little low. The National Bone Marrow Transplant Link points out that costs could run higher than $200,000, which might partially explain why some insurers are dropping the procedure from their plans (1999).

At IAT, June Austin takes all the initial calls from prospective patients or their family members. Her official title is patient coordinator, but for these callers she is a lifeline, providing common sense, comfort, and encouragement in her friendly American drawl. At the clinic, she's also the fixer, the maker of connections, the Gentle Enforcer. Well, maybe not so gentle.

One of the patients didn't turn up for his blood pull and serum for two days in a row. Clinic staff were concerned; phone calls were put through to his apartment, but there was no answer. The third day, Roy turned up unconcerned and popped his head through June's always open office door.

She pulled off her telephone head set: "Where the hell have you been, Roy? We've been worried."

"Cuba."

"Cuba? Why did you go to Cuba?"

Roy: "My friends were going. They invited me along. We went to Havana—it was a great trip. . . ."

June: "Now just wait a damn minute here, Roy. You are a patient at the IAT Clinic. You don't just go running off in the middle of treatment—to Cuba." Her voice grew steely. "You stay right here, you take your treatment, then at the end of your stay here, then you go to Cuba, or Tahiti, or Timbuktu if you want." Her perfectly manicured nails rapped the desk, punctuating her words. "You've got cancer for godsake. You're probably over there smoking cigars and messing with booze—OK, you do that if you want—AFTER YOU'VE FINISHED YOUR TREATMENT. Get it?"

A very chastened Roy: "I'm sorry June, I didn't think the clinic would mind."

June: "We mind, Roy, we mind. What the hell do you think we're here for? The good of our own health? No darlin', for the good of *your* health."

June is from Vermont—born and raised in the cold winters of that state, where people do not learn to pull punches. She lived for many years in Alabama before coming to the Bahamas, and the Alabama/Vermont combination makes June a unique species of steel magnolia. Beneath the soft southern overlay is an unwavering commitment to the people who come to the clinic; she reassures, cajoles, jokes, and scolds.

She is at the heart of the action while maintaining a watching brief, her perspective honed by the sharp certainty of her own faith and commitment to the clinic's work. She encourages patients to help each other, and heaven help anyone who balks. Of one young man who has been an IAT patient for twelve years, she says, "I asked him if I could give his name to prospective patients and he didn't want me to—I was so p.o.ed at him. I told him, 'We gave you a chance at more life, we gave you your life back, and you won't help others?' He's got to know we make sacrifices here to give people some life back to them; he has to, too. He said, 'But these people they talk for so long.' Of course they do, they're frightened, they need help and reassurance. I told him, 'We are all our brother's keepers, you know.'"

June says that her work at the clinic is almost like a calling. "I came for a visit in 1985," she says, "and I'm still here—fourteen years later."

So is her sister, as a patient. "When she was diagnosed with breast cancer, I told her to get right on down here, not to waste a minute on anything else," says June.

Dr. John Clement, the medical consultant for the clinic, was born and raised in Britain, and did his medical training at St. Thomas's Hospital in London, "the most prestigious hospital in the world," he grins, "or at least the most prestigious location—right opposite the British Houses of Parliament." He had a general practice in Dorset for five years before he started to apply for jobs in exotic places. "My wife, Jane, was game, the kids were young enough to be totally transportable. I applied for a job in Nassau. Didn't hear anything, so finally I phoned them. The reply was, 'Oh, that job's gone. But there's another in Freeport. Don't bother to look it up because it's not on the map yet. Interested?'"

He was. In 1965, Dr. Clement became the district medical officer for the Bahamian Ministry of Health on Grand Bahamas Island. He was following in the grand tradition of Evan Cottman, the famous Out Island Doctor, who in 1945 gave up school teaching in Madison, Indiana, to practice medicine from his boat among the Bahamian islands. Bahamians who had never seen a doctor in their lives came to him to "get sound." Dr. Clement treated patients at a clinic in Freeport, then hopped on his surgery bus and visited settlements around the island. After nine years of this, "It became pretty evident we were staying." He opened up a private practice in Freeport, which he maintains to this day.

When Lawrence Burton set up the IAT Clinic in 1977, he was allowed to employ two doctors licenced by the Bahamian authorities to practice medicine only as it pertained to the IAT program. He invited other local MDs to help out with patients' medical problems unrelated to the therapy. Dr. Clement was one of three who signed up.

"My whole family background is traditional medicine," Dr. Clement says. "My grandfather, my mother, my father, but we were very open-minded. Even back when I was in medical school, my sister was going to a homeopath. So when Burton asked for help, I was interested. When I saw what his serum was apparently doing for some people, I knew there was something in it."

It is obvious that Dr. Clement was born without blinkers, and never acquired them in his traditional medical education. "I saw people with the most incredible pathology, horrible, hopeless, and they were getting better at Burton's clinic."

Since Lawrence Burton's death in 1993, Dr. Clement has been acting as medical consultant. And cancer patients come from all over the world "to get sound."

Physically, the routine for IAT patients is perhaps inconvenient, but not taxing. It starts at 7:30 a.m. with the blood pull. (On occasion, if a patient is not well enough to attend the clinic, a doctor or staff member will go to his or her home to draw the blood.) Then breakfast, maybe with a few other patients at Mr. Baker's, a washed turquoise triple-domed mosque of a place housing a cafeteria and a shop. It is a landmark of sorts in the neighborhood, serving breakfast and lunch to office workers and IAT patients, dishing out peas with everything. The choice of chicken at lunchtime is broiled, barbecued, or baked. It all looks the same. Like very old Kentucky Fried pieces—and it's all delicious.

At about 9:30 a.m. everyone gathers back at the clinic to pick up their serum packets for the day. Laughter floats down the hall from the patients' waiting room. Laughter? Wait a minute—how could that be? Every person in that room carries within his or her body the most dread of diseases—cancer. And most carry within their heads a recent death sentence in the form of a flat, final statement from a doctor back home who has said, "We cannot do anything more for you." Or, "We have no treatment for your kind of cancer. I am sorry." Or, "Come back when you are in pain. We *can* manage the pain for you." With such a burden of illness and looming mortality, how can they be laughing?

The waiting room is like no other medical waiting room I've ever seen. It's like a shipboard party in that room—and the ship is definitely not the *Titanic*. They are on a voyage together, riding through a sea which is their disease; their ship of life for the time they are at the clinic is captained by the medical consultant and staff; their hope comes in ampoules of serum and from each other—the tangible evidence of survival, the success stories, the legends of the IAT alumni—the miracle patients who have been coming back for seventeen, eighteen years after being given three or four months to live those many years ago. Their legends anchor the net of optimism buoying up the frightened, tentative newcomers.

Hundreds of patients cycle through this clinic each month; there are six to eight new patients a week plus returning patients, back for their three-month or six-month or yearly tune-ups. If these patients were cars, they'd be putting the new car dealers out of business.

Carl, a transplanted New Yorker, delivers the bundle of needles to each person. His wife was one of the first patients to attend the IAT Clinic more than twenty-one years ago. She is one of the legends, not just a story, but a touchstone living just down the road. "This is the best medicine," says one patient. "This is what gives you hope." Carl helps around the place, transports patients, and is a kind of general factotum, handing out the sera with a joke or instruction. The process takes about an hour and a half. And this is when the room rocks. Or laughs, or weeps. Or even sings.

On a typical morning, thirty or forty people gather, sounding like a cocktail party in full swing; but the cocktails are not vodka martinis but urea, distilled water, herbal tea. A few stalwarts drink the fairly hefty coffee from the urn that is on all morning. The outside door opens again and again. Patients and their husbands, wives, partners, children, or friends come in, chatting, making plans. A woman pushes her husband in a wheelchair which promptly tips over backward. This is obviously a new task for her, a new role for him. Other patients rush to help: "You alright!?"

"Fine. Now I have your attention," he announces, still on his back on the floor. "For my next act. . . ."

"Hey," someone calls out, "I missed that entrance; could you do it again?"

One of the patients, Earl Kruger from Montreal, shows me a note tucked in with his needles that morning—each patient received one—requesting that patients give themselves their injections in privacy. "That's because of that fellow over there," Earl says, pointing at Michael sitting opposite, looking innocent. Suddenly, Michael pulls up his shirt, grabs a roll of flesh, plunges the needle in, and groans loudly. It is an act he does with great glee in public, and apparently someone complained. Michael has colon cancer with metastasis to the liver. Carl interjects, "I think he's got mets to the brain too." Michael grins. "Not yet," he says.

The affection, the humor, they are the coin of this place. Michael had gone to the Meridien Clinic in Tijuana and tried the Gerson therapy. "I drank fourteen juices a day, had five coffee enemas a day, strict vegetarian diet, lost thirty pounds, and after five months had another CAT scan and guess what, more spots on the liver." He came to IAT six weeks ago. "Here, they say eat, eat, so I eat and have gained back twenty pounds and joined the golf club."

The conversations cover the full gamut—jokes, tears, exchange of information, has anyone seen the doctor today? Hey, June is looking for you, didn't you pay your bill? There is much discussion about who is doing well, who isn't. The social life of the IAT patients on the island is constrained only by the limits of their energy and the need to carry their serum and needles with them always. They are insular to the extent that they rely heavily on one another for support, information, comfort, and fun.

"I have 'high tumor kill,'" says a new patient, reading the slip of paper tucked in with the bag of ampoules she's just been given. "Is that good or bad?" Several people answer her, giving reassurance, information, advice. Another waves a sheet of paper, announcing triumphantly, "Look, my test results are back from Miami—my blood counts are way better." Other patients cluster around, congratulating her.

There is chat, a joke is told, an anecdote related—"You have just arrived, haven't you? You should talk to Doris. She has only two weeks to live." Beat. "Hey, but that was seven years ago." Doris looks up, beaming proudly at the newcomer.

"OK, who's on for lunch today? My treat—I'm going home tomorrow, back to the real world. . . ."

There are tears, too. A patient sits hunched in a chair, hooked up to oxygen, waiting to see the doctor one more time before going to the airport and home . . . to die. Her cancer has outstripped the treatment, her immune system, her will. A young man meets a visiting oncologist in the hallway. "Doctor, it's not working. Nothing is working. Could I try more chemotherapy? Would you give it to me?" The oncologist is from the States, a caring, compassionate man who is searching everywhere for some therapy or combination of treatments that might work better than the status quo approaches. His own father died of pancreatic cancer. He takes the young man back with him to his clinic in the States, but the disease wins within a week.

Woolly Setteducato is back today. He's had a scare back home in New York. He had bad stomach aches—"How is that possible, Doc?" he said to his surgeon. "Don't forget I don't even *have* a stomach."

At his first surgery, the doctor had removed his entire stomach. Woolly had a heart condition as well, and the heart specialist had not expected that he would survive the operation. However, his options were not so great. If he didn't have the surgery, he wouldn't survive the cancer. He survived both. Woolly is seventy-two years old, bald, with a grey tufty tonsure, a face lined with laughter, and a short, strong body.

After the operation, the surgeon told Woolly's daughter that he didn't expect Woolly to survive for six months. That was two and a half years ago.

When an X-ray indicated that he had another tumor, apparently in the lung, Woolly says, "The surgeon told me, 'I gotta go in there, Woolly—I gotta see what it is.' He told me later he knew what it was; with my history of cancer, what else could it be. 'I was sure when I got in there I'd find you rotten with cancer.'"

The tumor, which was not in his lung but behind his heart—the heart that was supposed to have stopped beating years ago—was not a tumor but scar tissue.

No malignancy there. Woolly's wife, Ida, says, "[The surgeon] had Woolly open so he went through and turned over every organ like pages in a book. Clean. Absolutely clean. No cancer anywhere."

When Woolly came out of the anaesthetic and heard the good news, he thanked the surgeon. "Don't thank me," the doctor said. "Nothing to do with me. Thank those people in the Bahamas. They did it, not me. Get back as soon as you can."

Woolly and Ida are back for a month. But what a disaster. No beer, "I'm not allowed to drink." He pulls a sad face. "But not for ever," he adds hastily. "Just until I'm back on my feet."

It was Woolly who, on an earlier visit, turned the waiting room into a glee club. He came in with Ida, on their way to the airport. "I'm going home, goodbye, goodbye. I'll see you all in sixteen weeks," his voice boomed out over the chatter. "You know, the most beautiful people in the world come and go through that door, and we are all smiling. Don't forget that. And don't forget me." He burst into song then, "When you're smiling, when you're happy, the whole world smiles with you," and made his way around the room, saying goodbye to each person. "Help me, help me sing," he said, and soon wavery voices joined his, strengthening and shouting out the chorus. Everyone was indeed smiling, and there wasn't a dry eye in the place. The man is a life force, exuding strength and love and energy, enough to share with everyone there. "I'll see you all in April. Be there," he ordered, and turned to Ida, laughing, "They'll be glad to get rid of the old guy. . . ." The room was suddenly quiet as the door swung shut behind him.

"We will miss him," Seçkin said to no one in particular, her eyes dark with tears. "He makes us laugh. He makes Dave laugh."

Dave, her husband, is the one with advanced liver cancer who arrived at the clinic barely able to shuffle. He was the patient who said to me, as I walked through the waiting room, "Write a good book, write a good book about this place." His face was ashen, eyes sunken with illness and pain. He had been a big man, but now his flesh hung from a large bony frame. His stomach was swollen with disease, the skin of his feet and legs stretched and blotchy. Before cancer brought him down, he had been in control, a strong, confident consultant; staff did his bidding. And now there was a palpable air of bewilderment—his power could not budge the cancer cells. Suddenly he was at someone else's bidding, shoved ever downward by his illness and accepting direction from the clinic's doctors and the therapy program. A paradigm shift, he might have called it in the business jargon of his previous life.

When faced with the prospect of giving himself needles every hour or two of the day, he couldn't do it. "You must learn how, and give them to me," he told Seçkin. She gave him the first needle, and then said, "Now, you must learn. You must do it for yourself. . . ." His life had changed with such finality, with such speed. He sat in the clinic waiting room, watching quietly, studying how to live in his new world.

One month later, this same man sits joking about the urea he and other liver cancer patients drink each day. "It makes me so angry," he says. "You know, back in the days of Hippocrates, this was a common therapy—urea. When modern medicine turned chemical this kind of approach was pushed aside. But it works."

The idea is revolting to most people. To many conventional doctors, it is total nonsense. To a growing number of liver cancer patients it is the elixir of extended life. Dave holds up the disposable cup. "This is my cocktail now," he grins. "And my cocktail hour lasts the whole day. It tastes terrible— I think it's pure horse's pee." He cheerfully knocks it back. Because maybe, along with the injections he now gives himself every day, this is why his stomach is not as swollen, why he is not the livid yellow he was on arrival at the clinic, why the pain in his legs has nearly disappeared. Maybe it is why he can eat again, even walk a little on the beach. Maybe it's being away from the stress of the "real world." Maybe it's the sun and sea breezes. Or maybe it's the other patients, like Woolly Setteducato, who injected that whole room with hope and laughter. The immune systems did well that day.

The patients at IAT create their own, natural, unregulated support system. In their isolation from home, in the common bond of their disease, they become each other's family. The clinic is like the Gloucester pub in *The Perfect Storm*, where the sailors hung out waiting to go back out to sea: "the Crow's Nest . . . takes people in, gives them a place, loans them a family" (Junger 1997, p. 18).

4

The Immuno-Augmentative Therapy Clinic, Part II

The family atmosphere of the IAT Clinic is a by-product rather than a direct service of the clinic. It certainly wasn't one of the objectives of the founder, who from all accounts was not the fatherly type. Lawrence Burton was abrasive, childish, and unpredictable; he was also brilliant, caring, and utterly committed to his work. Howard Burton describes his father as "amicable, emotional, dedicated." His critics describe him as an arrogant quack. The patients who flocked to his clinic adored him. "He had a nasty personality, but I loved him," says Faye Pennington. Diagnosed at the age of forty-three with a non-Hodgkin's lymphoma, she had radiation and chemotherapy, neither of which slowed down her cancer. "I had it all over. It was in the bone marrow and really all over, even in my face. I had [a growth] right here, it was just a bag hanging off my face." Her doctor spoke about her prognosis then as "a matter of time." "He said to me, 'We are just going to make you as comfortable as we can for the time you have left.' That was in June 1982." Faye did not wait around to be made comfortable, but flew to Freeport instead. That was eighteen years ago. For Faye Pennington, Dr. Burton had given new meaning to the phrase "a matter of time."

When she arrived at the IAT Clinic, barely able to walk, pretty well without hope, Burton told her, "What you have is no more than a common cold."

"Can you imagine, after what they had told me in the States, when someone tells you that you have no more than a common cold? . . . What he told me, that helped me more than treatment. At the time if I could just have laid down and forgot it all . . . I didn't care if I died. . . . I guess that I had gotten to the point that nothing mattered to me anymore. When he told me that, it gave me something to live for . . . I hadn't had one doctor give me any good news. And for him to give me that good news, it completely turned my world around. After he told me that, I might have doubts for a minute or two minutes, whereas before I didn't have hope except for a minute or two minutes."

Faye credits God and Burton—in that order—for her survival over cancer. "By the Lord sending me here, it turned my whole world around. He can work miracles through different people. Dr. Burton was not a believer but he didn't have to be. I think the Lord can anoint an infidel. . . ."

"One of the things I loved about him," another patient says: "He could be ornery, real ornery, but he told it like it was. He was honest and upfront and did not watch his words."

Apparently not. "I just told off a bitch of a know-it-all TV reporter from Manhattan. I told her that her family deserved dying of cancer because they didn't have enough sense to look for my therapy. . . . I don't need this shit anymore . . . I can go to Europe, or I can close the door and live very comfortably for my remaining years" (Burton quoted in Null and Steinman 1986, p. 106).

Dr. Clement says, "I got on very well with Burton. He could be a miserable SOB but I liked him." The first time my wife met him, she came away from his house and grabbed my arm, exclaiming, "He exists, he exists!" "Who exists? Of course he exists. I'm working for the old bugger. . . ." "No, I mean Professor Brainstorm—he exists. He is Burton." (Brainstorm was a comic-strip character in Britain, hair on end, ideas and inventions exploding from a teeming brain.)

Burton was a chameleon, but only in the eyes of his beholders. His underlying color was a single-minded focus on his patients and on his research. He had little time for the social niceties. He didn't play by the rules—he didn't *know* the rules. Some time after his term in office, U.S. President Jimmy Carter came to see Burton when his sister got cancer. Dr. Clement relates the story: "We had supper, we showed him around the clinic and when Carter's car came for him I called to Burton, 'Mr. Carter is leaving now.'

"Burton was already back at his desk. He looked up, said, 'Oh OK. 'Bye, Jimmy. You're a good guy, Jimmy. I'll vote for you next time.' And went right back to his work."

His patients might have loved him, but the medical establishment pretty much hated him. The feeling was mutual. "The [medical] establishment believes the accepted treatment should take precedence over the health of the patient. This is acceptable for allergies and ingrown toenails, but not for cancer. These doctors favor status quo. In cancer, that means death" (Burton quoted in Wright 1985, p. 46).

The National Cancer Institute (NCI), the National Institutes for Health (NIH), the American Cancer Society (ACS), the Food and Drug Administration (FDA), the Sloan-Kettering

Institute for Cancer Research (S.-K.)—he took them all on in the end. It was the battle of Burton versus the Acronyms. To his supporters it was David against Goliath, but without quite the same outcome. To his kinder critics it was Quixote tilting at windmills. And to his sworn enemies—the high priests of medical science, as they are sometimes described—it was a righteous crusade against the infidel, a crusade that lasted decades and boiled over borders.

Born in the Bronx in 1926, Burton studied at Brooklyn College and New York University, where he earned his Ph.D. in biology in 1955. For the next fifteen years he worked in the field of cancer research at the California Institute of Technology, New York University, and St. Vincent's Hospital, where he was senior investigator in the Hodgkin's Disease Research Laboratory (Moss 1996, p. 236). Other sources have him as senior oncologist at St. Vincent's, an unlikely position for someone without a medical degree. This claim—perhaps wishful thinking on the part of one of his defenders—may have been the source of his detractors' more serious invective about his credentials. Not only was he not a medical doctor, he wasn't even a horse doctor, huffed the *New York Daily News* in early 1986. His therapy was nothing more than "snake-oil" gimmickry, a rip-off engineered by a zoologist (Null and Steinman 1986). That Burton himself never claimed to be anything other than a researcher did not stop his critics from heaping scorn on him for not being what he never claimed to be.

While working at St. Vincent's in the late 1950s, Burton and a team of researchers, including Frank Friedman, Antonio Rottino, M.L. Kaplan, and Robert Kassel, managed to extract from mouse blood a factor that caused long-term remission of cancer in mice. This indeed was a breakthrough. "The animals' cancers would begin, in a matter of hours, to *disappear*" (Moss 1996, p. 237). There was even more excitement when the team subsequently found that the tumor-inhibiting factor could cross species lines: a factor derived from mouse blood could trigger anticancer effects in human cells, a finding that suggested that such an approach would work as well with humans as with mice.

At this point, in the early 1960s, the team had grants from both the National Cancer Institute and the Damon Runyon Memorial Fund for Cancer Research. The five men were optimistic; there was excitement about their discoveries; the future looked rosy for both them and their research.

Enter the Sloan-Kettering Institute (S.-K.). Interested in the research of Burton and his colleagues, S.-K. sent Dr. John Harris to check them out. After several months of working together, Burton, Friedman, and Harris published a paper, "Synergistic Action of Two Refined Leukemic Tissue Extracts in Oncolysis of Spontaneous Tumors," in the *Transactions of the New York Academy of Sciences*, on which Harris's name came after those of the original researchers. Not acceptable. The director of the Sloan-Kettering Institute told Harris that S.-K. scientists never allowed their names to be listed after those of scientists of "lesser" institutions (Moss 1996, p. 237). "In those days," Dr. Harris would say later, "S.-K. always wanted to come out playing first trumpet, no matter who wrote the tune. When the director sent me down to St. Vincent's, the idea was for me to smuggle back as much information as I could. I didn't go for that, and Friedman, Burton and I published everything that went on. This got disapproval back at [Sloan-Kettering]" (Anderson 1974, p. 45).

From this petty skirmish, the lines for a much bigger battle were drawn. After contract negotiations with Sloan-Kettering fell through, all Burton's funding was suddenly terminated. The story now becomes a free-for-all of accusations and counter-accusations, innuendos, half-truths and, apparently, outright lies.

The team reapplied for government grants, and their applications were turned down on the advice of "a Sloan-Kettering chemotherapist who was sent to make a site visit for the National Cancer Institute" (Moss 1996, p. 238). Burton had shaken his fist under the nose of one establishment organization and ended up taking them all on. It was not a wise career move.

Meanwhile, the team kept working, this time with mice with spontaneous breast cancers. More exciting developments: when these mice were injected with the mouse-derived tumor-inhibiting factor, their tumors appeared to melt away. "It was dramatic to see how the tumor would undergo necrosis. . . . That is important, and it is something very fundamental that should be studied," said one of the team members, Dr. Rottino, described by Ralph Moss as "a scholarly research physician not given to overstatement" (ibid., p. 238).

In 1966, Burton and Friedman were invited to give a demonstration of their findings at the annual American Cancer Society Science Writers' Seminar in Phoenix, Arizona. In front of a group of prominent scientists and reporters, they injected the tumor deblocking agent into four mice with large tumors. A few hours later, the massive tumors had virtually disappeared.

The response was immediate and mixed; some of the audience were disbelieving, claiming the mice had been switched; others were completely convinced that Burton and his colleagues had taken a huge step toward successful treatment of cancer. Ironically, it was the reaction of Burton's supporters that seems to have helped launch him on his journey beyond the pale of the medical establishment. That evening, newspapers across the country carried headlines about the experiment, including one that trumpeted: "15-minute cancer cure for mice: humans next?" The expectations were set—too high. Within a year, when Burton repeated his experiment for the New York Academy of Science, with the same amazing results, many of his peers insisted that it was a trick. Burton lashed out publicly at his detractors, collecting more enemies in high places.

At first, though, it appeared that Burton and Friedman were on their way again. The American Cancer Society approached them about a grant, but Burton felt there were too many strings attached. They were asked to change the wording of their proposal to match the wording to language "everyone can understand," the ACS told them, such as "antibody" and "antigen." Burton refused: "It would have been dishonest to use those terms without being sure of exactly what we were dealing with. They wanted us to label unknowns" (Anderson 1974, p. 46). The ACS also told them that their project was getting too big for just two men. If they would give it to a more established lab, the ACS would give the two of them a one-year contract of $15,000. Burton's response was a furious rejection: "We should give someone all our data for one year's salary for one man, and no assurance of a job after that?" (ibid., p. 46).

In 1974, Burton and Freidman left St. Vincent's and with private financial support opened the Immunology Research Foundation in Great Neck, Long Island. Medical doctors affiliated with the foundation began to treat cancer patients with Burton's blood proteins.

That same year, *New York* magazine ran a story on Burton and Friedman, entitled "The Politics of Cancer—How do You Get the Medical Establishment to Listen?" Over the next few years, the medical establishment did pay attention, but as a horse does to flies, flicking irritably in the apparent hope that they would buzz off.

Within the next three years, they both did, but in different directions. In 1975, Burton and Friedman filed for patents covering the three proteins they were using and their methods of extraction. These were granted. At this point, Sloan-Kettering re-entered the picture. Apparently, it even sent a few patients to Burton's clinic (Moss 1996, p. 241), and Burton and Freidman, encouraged by this change of heart among the establishment leaders, applied for an Investigational New Drug (IND) permit from the Food and Drug Administration which would have allowed them to conduct human tests of their treatment. It was not to happen.

Dr. William Terry and other NCI officials made a short on-site visit to Burton's laboratory at Great Neck. The visit was not a success. Dr. Terry later claimed that there was no evidence that anything was happening at Burton's clinic. And Burton claimed that Dr. Terry was "the most antagonistic SOB I've ever met."

This about set the stage for any future interaction between Burton on one side and the Acronym Big Guns on the other: the NCI, the ACS, the NIH, the S.-K., and the FDA.

Burton's IND application foundered on the shoals of bureaucratic red tape and his inability to provide certain information, for instance, the LD-50 (lethal dose) of his treatment (that is, how much would it take to kill 50 percent of the test mice, a standard test required before a treatment is judged to be safe for humans). This was a tough one, since there *was* no lethal dose. Burton's team "would be happy to oblige," as one of them said, except that there were no toxic effects from the serum, whatever the dose. They could not kill any of the mice unless they diluted the serum to such an extent that it would be the water killing the animals and not the fractions.

Another requirement was that patients could be treated with a new experimental drug only after they had exhausted all conventional treatments. What usually happened was that the conventional treatments exhausted the patients first. Burton objected strenuously to this demand.

After almost two years of trying to answer the barrage of FDA questions and still not receiving permission to treat human cancer patients, Burton and Friedman withdrew their application in exasperation at what they perceived as personal and professional jealousies, a medical status quo determined to squash the little guys, and an unfair funding and regulatory system. Friedman gave up altogether, and Burton moved his clinic to the Bahamas where he was given permission to treat patients with his therapy. True to form, Burton told his first batch of patients at his new clinic in Freeport, "You may be wasting some time, but most of you came after you had wasted all your time" (Wright 1985, p. 32). In 1977 and 1978 one in five of Burton's patients improved and went home; no small miracle considering the serious condition of most of those treated.

The majority of early successes were claimed in malignant melanoma, head and neck, bladder, colon, and prostate cancers. It seemed that Burton was being proven right when he said that "patients would do better outside the country where conventional treatment would not be prerequisite to receiving immuno-augmentative therapy" (ibid., p. 29).

Many patients have done just that over the intervening

twenty-two years, flourishing on the therapy, and on not only the support, but the survival of other patients.

For Canadians, Americans, and Europeans there is an incongruity about cancer in the subtropics—how can such an ugly mutant survive the beauty, the warm sea breezes, the ambling pace of the Bahamas? At the IAT Clinic, there is no question, the setting helps. In fact, the sublime climate works its way into criticisms of the clinic: Who wouldn't feel better sitting on a beach for three months carved out of the stress and worries of the daily routine back home?

The IAT Clinic has other perks, not least the humane and undidactic attitudes of the clinic staff, exemplified in the patient-orientation sessions held every two or three weeks by Dr. Clement, and the self-injection training classes conducted by Lynn Austin, a registered nurse who has worked at the clinic since its earliest days. She has weathered its storms of closure and censure with a calm good humor. For the new patients, giving themselves injections is a daunting prospect. Lynn shows them how, reassures, makes them laugh. In a matter of days, most are as confident as nurses, swabbing and jabbing their own flesh. "Can't feel it, not even a pin prick," most say. It is practical, daily evidence that they have taken control—no longer slaves to someone else's medical schedule. "I've never felt so free in my life," says Steve.

At the orientation session for newcomers, the patients and their partners—wives, husbands, friends—sit around the table. Some are apprehensive, some frightened, some resigned, some belligerent. Most write down every word Dr. Clement utters. A few sit back with a glazed look of incomprehension. Some have been doing the rounds of the alternative therapy clinics and have stopped computing. Others have simply been short-circuited by the fear and pain of their disease. It is here that Dr.

Clement's good humor and good sense become obvious. He shows a cheerful disregard for factors that seem less important than the therapy (for instance, instructions in the print material handed out to the patients slightly contradict what he has to say about diet—"Well, I think a little red meat is OK if it's well cooked." He looks a bit bemused at the shocked response from a couple of the patients. "Just eat healthily," he says. In other words, don't obsess.

He reassures patients with information, with empathy, with humor. "There are two doctors here every day. Ask, and you can see them anytime, not just on your pre-booked appointment. And you can fill in a form any day about how you are, or if you have questions. We need these, it's a good means of communication. We look at these every day, so ask anything." Pause. "Anything medically relevant, that is. I don't give stock tips."

What he does give patients is something far more valuable, a viable medical therapy that bolsters the body's ability to fight some cancers—and hope.

This is re-enforced by the powerful message patients receive when they learn that family members of the medical consultant, the patient coordinator, and the clinic administrator are IAT patients. It would be hard to find a clearer endorsement of the staff's own belief in the therapy.

Dr. Clement's sister, Janet Lang, started on immuno-augmentative therapy in 1983, after a diagnosis of breast cancer and a radical mastectomy at the age of forty-seven. "The treatment people were having at home [Britain] wasn't that brilliant. I mean, many people who had had mastectomies years ago and nothing further, hardly any are still alive, and for those who had radiation, it did a lot of damage. . . . There was a lot of pressure for me to have [further treatment], but I spoke to John—Dr. Clement—and he said, 'Don't, you won't lose anything by coming out here. Are you prepared to come straight out?' I had confidence in an older brother who just made me feel OK in a way that the doctors [at home] hadn't. I did have a very nice GP but he said, "Well, you might have five years, you could have ten . . . um . . . we don't know.' The hospital [where she'd had her surgery] was doing a study of various treatments for people with cancer so I was a control I suppose, because I was going to have nothing as far as they were concerned." Janet was on IAT for eight and a half years. She still comes back to the Bahamas once a year for a tune-up, now seventeen years after her diagnosis.

The clinic administrator, Edmund Granger, was a "city boy," as he describes himself, from Nassau where at the age of eighteen he went to work for Batelco, the Bahamian telephone company. He retired forty-four years later as head of operations in Freeport. That was in 1983. Unlike the usual horror stories about people who, within a few weeks of retirement, get sick and die, Granger's story has a cruel twist. After his retirement, it was his wife who died. When diagnosed with breast cancer, she had a mastectomy "which got it all," so much so that it was deemed that she needed no further treatment.

"I'd had three months of retirement and that was enough of that. I had just started at the clinic when my wife got sick again. But those were early days for me at IAT, I didn't know very much about the place, and felt obliged to accept my wife's doctor's advice." Which was to go to Miami for radiation treatments. She died shortly after.

But even before this, cancer had gnawed its way into the Granger family in the most unforgivable way of all. His daughter was twenty-six years old, back home after a vacation in England. "She was suffering from stomach pain," Ed Granger says, his face so sad with memory. "It was severe and persistent enough that after tests showed nothing, it was decided to do an exploratory operation. She was full of cancer." The liver was the primary site, everything else was the secondary. They closed her up. She died within three months.

Edmund Granger must have to wonder if he is being stalked by the disease. His second wife, Gena, had a scar on her shin, the result of a water-skiing accident twenty years before. The scar seemed to be enlarging. It was melanoma. After the operation to remove it, the surgeon in the United States told her that they'd got it all, and there was no need for further treatment. Wrong. Gena is on IAT treatment now, has been for three years, is working hard and feeling fine. "Your quality of life is about 9000 percent better here," she says, "and you just assimilate the needles into your life. You know, when you consider that most of the people who come here have one foot in the grave, what an incredible success story the clinic is."

June Austin puts it another way. "Remember, we get bodies here." She's not being callous, just realistic.

"You know, something works here. Through conventional medical eyes, it looks very primitive, and how much is the serum I'm not 100 percent sure. But . . . here, you get your psyche topped up . . . the patients believe in each other, they believe in the serum, they were nearly dead when they came here, most of them, they'd been rejected, they were cancer rejects of the system and they come here and they're not rejected anymore . . . it's an attitude, you walk in the door and you look around at everyone and you think, 'He's got a miracle, she's got a miracle, and I'm going to get one too . . . it's a wonderful place.'"

In December 1998, a German doctor visited the IAT Clinic; she had been sent to check it out because of plans to reopen a clinic in Germany that uses IAT protocols and approach. She was very thorough, studied patient records, observed lab and computer processes, puzzled over all the licencing documentation allowing the clinic to operate. She was particularly interested in "three-month response rates" of patients, the standard staging observation in clinical studies: how much tumor shrinkage, patient weight gain, toxic side effects, and so on. Dr. Clement explained that IAT doesn't work that way: it is not a frontal attack on the tumor, so such standards can't be applied with any accuracy. The German doctor was doubtful. Finally, Dr. Clement called to a patient he saw in the waiting room.

"Michelle, come and meet Dr. X from Germany. Could you tell her about your situation, what cancer you have, and how you are doing?"

"I have renal cell cancer," Michelle said cheerfully.

"For how long you have had it?" the doctor asked.

"Seventeen years."

"Then you are cured?"

"Well, I have metastasis to the liver. And to the lung."

"Then you are not cured. For how long have you had these metastases?"

"Seventeen years."

Finally, Dr. Clement says, there is a glimmer of understanding. Michelle has lived with her cancer for seventeen years. Emphasis on "lived."

One morning, in the IAT patient waiting room I am chatting with Marcia and Mike while they wait for their serum.

Mike: Great earrings. I have to buy those earrings.

Marcia: For me, for me—I love those earrings.

Mike: And she wants that skirt too.

Another patient: Well I like those shoes, can I have the shoes?

A fourth patient chimes in: I kind of like her hair. . . .

I twirl in the middle of the room: Hey, nobody want my T-shirt? What's wrong with my T-shirt?

Mike: Wrong words on it.

Hennessey, one of the office staff, says, "No, no one wants your shirt 'cause the labels are all hanging off it." She tucks the labels back in.

At the end of the room a new patient sits, first day here: a few minutes earlier she had been in the hallway with her husband, weeping and weeping. He rubbed her back, trying to console her. She looks so ill, unable to walk without a walker, her legs like sticks, her body emaciated. She is a young woman, in her late thirties, her face already ravaged with suffering. But at this small gust of silliness, she looks up, gently sitting straighter, a small smile starting, her eyes a little brighter, no longer weeping. The spirit in that room is starting to do its work. Hope and faith are powerful antidotes.

But the actual therapy, does *it* work? The definitive answer is Yes. No. Maybe. Sometimes.

This would be the only honest answer for most cancer therapies: does chemo work? Does radiation? Does a fat-free diet and detoxification? Do mega-vitamins? Shark cartilage and essiac tea? The new cancer vaccines? It depends on what you mean by "work," how you define success. There are the statistical successes based on probabilities—stats say that women with stage 1 breast cancer, no nodes positive, have a 90 percent chance of survival for five years, but your mother or sister or daughter is in the 10 percent who doesn't make it. For her, the treatment did not work, was not successful. It depends on whether "success" is defined as longer life or better quality of life; depends on the definition of "cure"—five-year survival? Eight years? Sixteen? It depends on the specific cancer being treated, depends on how the "evidence" is defined, analyzed, and categorized.

And it depends on whom you ask. An epidemiologist will answer in statistics. Feeling better does not figure in epidemiology. Getting better is translated into population figures. A medical oncologist will answer in statistics related to specific therapy and cancer: chemo works for childhood leukemia. Feeling better is nice, but not necessarily a good symptom in chemotherapy. It might mean the doses are not high enough. According to the U.S. National Cancer Institute, this is a danger signal to watch for in alternative therapies: "Do those who endorse the treatment claim that it is harmless and painless and that it produces no unpleasant side effects? Because treatments for cancer must be very powerful, they frequently have unpleasant side effects (NCI web site, *www.betterhealth.com*). A patient will answer according to his or her own experience, a cohort of one, where feeling better is high on the measurement stick.

Back to the original question. Does immuno-augmentative therapy work?

In the summer of 1999, the IAT Clinic launched an independent scientific investigation of the serum, its make-up, and how it works. The microbiologist in charge says that, in a way, the IAT Clinic is a clinical trial in itself, where human beings have been taking the serum since the mid-1970s. The job of researchers now is to establish the scientific basis through animal studies. It is the scientific method turned on its head, working from human trials back through animal and in-vitro models to evaluate the biological effects of IAT sera on tumors.

A preliminary review of IAT's mesothelioma patients conducted in 1999 by the National Foundation for Alternative Medicine (NFAM) shows promising results. The longest recorded survival of any peritoneal mesothelioma patient that it could find in the published literature is ten years. The mean survival is 2.24 years. Two IAT patients included in the NFAM review are alive and functioning with disease well beyond that point; one has survived fifteen years and the other eighteen years. Another patient is still alive after twelve years, and several more are still alive many years beyond the mean survival rate.

An external survey of all IAT patients also carried out in 1999 found that the average survival was five years from diagnosis compared to the expected average survival of three years.

So does this mean that IAT works? "*Absolutely not,*" says Saul Green, Ph.D., in an article in *Journal of the American Medical Association* (JAMA) published in 1993. Retired from the Sloan-Kettering Institute, and now a private health consultant, he attacks immuno-augmentative therapy for being bad science. His research, funded by a National Cancer Institute grant, was based on "the author's search of the scientific literature, the written communications in the files of the Division of Cancer Treatment of the National Cancer Institute, proceedings of legal actions, minutes of public hearings, media publications, and patient information brochures" (Green 1993, p. 1723). He did not visit the clinic; he did not interview IAT medical staff or patients. He did not consider the "anecdotal" evidence of long-term survival of so many IAT patients. However, he still summarizes that

[Burton's] tumor complement fraction has no complement activity, his blocking protein has not been shown to block anything, his deblocking protein has not been shown to deblock anything, and his human tumor cells have never shown to lyse following the interaction of tumor antibody and tumor complement. Finally, since there is no information on the quality control procedures being used in the manufacture of the IAT materials, there is the possibility that they may be unsterile and, therefore, hazardous for use in humans (ibid.).

Green's lack of information on quality control procedures—given that he did no primary research—is curious grounds for finding Burton's clinic guilty of having none. Such blanket condemnation of immuno-augmentative therapy could be rooted in Green's well-documented rejection of immunology in any form as a cancer therapy: "The belief that the clinically normal human immune system maintains a continuous surveillance for cancer cells and can evoke an immunologic intervention to destroy them is so appealing and full of emotionally charged wishful thinking that it has become dogma in the lay literature" (ibid. 1993, p. 1719).

Notwithstanding Dr. Green's doubts, the whole field of immunotherapy is advancing into the mainstream. "In the last five years, biological therapies have joined the three traditional approaches of cancer therapy—surgery, radiation, and chemotherapy—in the effective treatment of cancer patients," says Steven A. Rosenberg, M.D., Ph.D., chief of the National Cancer Institute's (NCI) Surgery Branch. "Gene therapy and other immunotherapies represent the fourth approach to cancer treatment that is based on the immune system's ability to mount an attack on cancer" (National Cancer Institute [U.S.] 1999).

"*Absolutely yes*, IAT works" say the many IAT patients who were written off twelve, fifteen, seventeen, even twenty years ago but who are happily thriving now. They represent "anecdotal" evidence which is not acceptable in the court of medical science.

Dr. Marty Goldstein *knows* it works. For sixteen years he has been using Burton's immuno-augmentative therapy in his veterinary practice in the state of New York, but his "patients" come from all over the country. Dr. Goldstein reports that when he and his brother Bob, also a veterinarian, added IAT into their existing protocols for fighting cancer, they witnessed an almost tripled success rate in clinical improvement and actual tumor regression. And that's with no other variable added. "[IAT] also reversed 'patients' such as those blind and convulsing with CAT-scanned brain tumors. And these animals live in Brooklyn. . . . Lots of people criticize IAT, saying it's nothing more than a placebo, that patients feel better on it because they are in the sun and sand on a beautiful warm island away from all their daily worries. They come back home, and wham, they're sick again. Well, there's not much sun and sand during Brooklyn winters."

"*Maybe* IAT works," say a growing number of researchers working in the field of immunology, including doctors and chemists from Europe and North American immunologists who are applying scientific research criteria to study the efficacy of IAT.

One immunologist points out that although the case for IAT treatment has been used clinically for more than twenty years, the preclinical phase of testing was never published. Critics say this was because there was nothing to publish; defenders say it was because the medical journals closed ranks and refused to touch any of Burton's work. Without those preclinical results it has been difficult for immunologists and microbiologists to evaluate just what is happening.

Once more, cancer patients are in the middle—whom to believe? Peter Frank's wife, Marcia, chose IAT, but it was not an easy decision. His anguished comment could apply not just to alternative therapies, but to many therapies: "It is the treachery of cancer treatment—so many people out there offering treatment. Who is a fraud? Who is real? To know where to go is so difficult."

5

Hocus-Pocus or Healing? The Mexican Tour, Part I

Like it or not, patients are increasingly finding themselves in the role of decision maker in their own cancer treatment. It is a bewildering and awesome burden, especially in the alternative therapy world where there are few signposts, few guides, and even fewer standards against which to measure them. So many alternative therapy centers sit on the banks of the mainstream. A huge challenge for cancer patients is to find accurate and balanced information solid enough to support what could be a life and death—and expensive—decision.

Mostly, you hear of an alternative therapy by word of mouth: a sister-in-law, a cousin, a friend of a friend has been to a clinic in Mexico or Germany, a centre in Britain, a hospital in Switzerland, Santo Domingo, or Texas—and has done well on iscador, meditation, magnets, laetrile, diets, or vaccines. Then you set out to find out more. You might go to the Internet, where you'll find information, certainly, but how helpful is it? The sources completely contradict each other: the

Quackwatch site, for instance, pretty well trashes all alternative cancer treatment centers, therapies, and practitioners. The alternative medicine sites pretty much support them all. You can find books and occasionally a video on these centers, but there are few that don't take sides, building their case upon vested interests. Or you can visit the clinic or center, to try and assess for yourself whether you want to entrust your health, possibly your life, to the people you meet there.

I had heard only passing mention of the Immuno-Augmentative Therapy Clinic before going to Freeport on holiday. A casual beach chat with an IAT patient was the launch for years of research, interviewing, and investigation. During this time, I talked to patients and staff, studied medical records, and spent time in the computer room, the lab, and the waiting room at the clinic. Such access has provided a strong base from which to observe and comment on IAT, to hear the patients' stories, to focus on the issues around alternative cancer therapies in general. Against that backdrop, I also visited other alternative cancer treatment centers, but as a prospective patient might, someone without the luxury of time, someone having to decide quickly on a treatment to arrest active disease. It was a daunting experience.

When you start exploring the world of alternative cancer therapy clinics, likely you will hear first of the Mexican clinics, especially those in Tijuana. And mostly what you will hear will not be complimentary. Before you make a decision about treatment at any of these centers, you can take a bus tour to visit them all, sort of like a factory outlet tour of cancer deals.

The United States wears a skirt of these cancer treatment centres around its borders, just beyond reach of the regulatory authorities that rule medical practices within the country. In Tijuana, Mexico, a nest of them flourish. Linked, on the surface, by the common bond of exile and a broadly similar philosophical approach to treatment, these establishments have prospered, waned, and prospered again in the tawdry streets of a city that spreads up to the U.S. border like a rash. The border is easy to cross from the States. You walk through rusty ten-foot turnstiles, or drive past customs and immigration with a congestion of cars carrying party-seekers and tourists. Like so many border towns, it attracts borderline activities. Pretty much anything goes in Tijuana.

Though it is easy to get into Mexico through this border crossing, getting back into the States is not so easy. Cars and buses are checked thoroughly for aliens; the dogs trained to sniff out people and drugs wait to be called into action— which they are several times in a night. Cancer patients see little of this as they cross the border, their vision tunneled into a focus on finding a therapy that will reverse the death sentence they have received from the doctors back home.

The Cancer Control Society, which operates out of Los Angeles, California, runs tours to these clinics. Instead of hitting the market stalls in search of a bargain, the riders on its buses are looking to buy a miracle.

It is an unlikely setting for miracles. Or maybe not. But for new arrivals, the atmosphere is unsettling, discouraging; it sets off alarm bells. Everyone in this border town seems to be on the make, so why not the clinics? In a five-minute walk from the border to the euphemistically named visitor's center—not a soul knew where it was—street vendors and taxi drivers offered me a range of services.

"Taxi, lady? Where you wanna go? I know Tijuana. I take you on tour."

"Lady! Lady! Jewellery, lady? Pure silver, cheap. Best bargain. Walk with me now."

"Bad teeth, lady?"

What??

"You got bad teeth, bad teeth?" A young woman hands me a flyer advertising a dentist.

The border area throngs with pharmacies all advertising drugs at 40, 50, 70 percent off American prices. Don't have a prescription? You can buy that too.

For many people attending the clinics within Mexico as outpatients, home for that time is a motel on the U.S. side of the border. The rooms are clean and there is a special rate for cancer patients. But it is a place where the desk clerk gives you the TV remote with your key when you check in, the empty shampoo/soap dispenser hangs crookedly from the bathroom wall, and the window air-conditioners bleed dirty rivulets of water across the pavement in front of the rooms. The vista is parking lot and fast food: Taco Bell, McDonald's, Coco's, and Denny's belch out their greasy aroma.

Three patients sit on a bench outside the hotel lobby waiting for the shuttle bus to one of the clinics across the border. A woman, from New York, holds a large envelope marked BONE: her X-rays from a hospital back home. "I've been coming here since 1984. That's when I was diagnosed with breast cancer. I stay in this hotel for a week each time I come down, only twice a year now. I have to do this because our dear FDA won't let us have three of the drugs I get from American Biologics. Why not? They've helped so many of us. But we have to come down and stay here, crossing the border each day, like . . . I don't know, like criminals."

You question how you have come to this place, both geographically and in your life. Arthur Barr and his sister, Judy, have come from Nebraska. "Yesterday, I just wanted to turn around and go home," Arthur says. We are sitting in the garden of the first clinic on the Cancer Control Society tour. At least we hoped it is the first. We thought we had been missed at our pickup points by the bus and so had taken cabs through the Tijuana gridlock to the clinic in hopes of connecting with the tour. It turned out we hadn't been missed at all. It was merely our northern impatience not adjusted yet to our new time zone—*mañana* time. A fair amount of good-natured astonishment greeted our assumption that 9:30 meant 9:30. By the end of the day the bus was running four hours late.

The Cancer Control Society came into being in 1963 as the International Association of Cancer Victims and Friends, Inc. Following her diagnosis of breast cancer in 1959, the association's founder, Cecile Pollock Hoffman, had a mastectomy and three years later, an oophorectomy (removal of ovaries) to slow down extensive bone metastasis. It didn't work. The Tumor Board of her local hospital in San Diego advised her to have her pituitary gland removed. Instead she went to Montreal where in May 1963 she started laetrile therapy with the McNaughton Foundation. "I improved noticeably and at once." Her doctor in San Diego agreed to administer the substance even though it was banned in the States but then was advised by his lawyer that if he did he would lose his licence. Hoffman finally turned to Dr. Ernesto Contreras in Tijuana, closer to home, to continue the treatment.

"Riding to Tijuana daily, my mind said: Organize—organize—organize. . . . And since I had to go to Montreal, then to Tijuana—two foreign cities—to fight for my life, the organization must be international" (Cancer Control Society).

In 1973, the Cancer Control Society took its present name when it became an educational, non-profit California corporation.

There are forty-two people on today's tour, including a group of nurses from the Los Angeles area. The tour and a weekend conference on alternative cancer therapies are part of a credit in a continuing education program. "I don't know why everyone thinks that is so unusual," one nurse says. "We want to learn about other cancer treatments too, not just the ones we work with at home." The rest of the passengers are cancer patients, their companions . . . and people who are planning ahead. "Before disease strikes . . . discover your options," says the Cancer Control Society information sheet.

One gleamingly healthy woman (perfect hair, perfect teeth) said proudly, "Oh, I've never had cancer. But when I get it, I'll know what to do." "When" not "if." The spectrum of bus riders provides a complete sounding board, ranging from skeptics to fervent believers, from open-minded observers to people who are simply here for the beer. In this case, the beer is carrot juice. And then there are the people who are not here for a credit or information to store away against the future. They need to know about treatments now, not tomorrow, because cancer has already struck.

Arthur and his sister Judy are here because of Arthur's seven-year-old daughter, Leslie. She had fallen off her new bike two weeks earlier and broken her arm. Then the nightmare began. X-rays and tests indicated more than a broken arm—much, much more. It was Ewing's sarcoma, a fearsome, fast-moving children's cancer, already settled in the bone of her upper arm. Arthur has a picture of her—an impish face with a grin that would melt ice, long black hair shining with health. "Her hair is already falling out with the chemo," he says, his eyes blank with pain. His wife was back in Nebraska with Leslie who was in hospital after her first chemo treatment. She had also developed a Staphylococcus infection from the portacath implant.

"She went down so fast with that first chemo," Arthur says. "How can we do this to her again? And again? She trusts us to make her better, not sicker . . . I don't agree with the theory behind chemo. It doesn't make sense to attack the body with a treatment. It makes sense to help the body fight disease."

They had come to see if any of these clinics might support that logic.

The American Biologics Hospital where we waited is set back behind a small walled patio on a narrow side street, not far from one of Tijuana's two bull rings. A stone fountain gurgles in the corner; a couple of patients sit under a shade tree in the dappled sun. An ambulance pulls into the short steep driveway to deliver a patient on a stretcher.

The tour bus finally puts in its appearance, edging down the cramped street like a big, white whale slowly beaching itself in the shallows. The driver is obviously used to the rigors of driving an oversized luxury bus down the tiny byways of an urban maze originally used by nothing bigger than a donkey. The passengers climb down and we join them for the tour of the clinic, a modern, spanking clean, two-story structure tucked in among the sun-crumbled walls of older, poorer buildings crowding the block. Street space is at a premium; the narrow entrance to the clinic belies the spacious interior.

The medical director, Dr. Rodrigo Rodríguez, speaks to our group on a walled upstairs terrace, a warm and welcoming expanse of burnt-sienna tiles, baking sun, and shade umbrellas hovering above the fumes and roar of truck traffic below. The terrace opens off the treatment room, an airy pleasant space, with windows all along one side, leather recliners in a big circle, and a TV set showing a wildlife program on hyenas. It is hard to resist the siren call of the easy metaphor: desperate and ill, patients come to these clinics for help, only to be devoured by the quacks waiting like the hyenas to feed on that desperation. This is certainly the medical establishment's "take" on the Tijuana clinics.

Melody Leonardi sits in one of the recliners, her long, reddish-blonde hair framing rosy cheeks and bright eyes, the picture of health if you overlook the intravenous line running into her arm. And the brightness of her eyes is caused by tears as she talks about her three-year-old daughter back home. "I've got to be here for her. I can't leave her. I've got to beat this thing. I'm going to beat this disease." She was diagnosed with non–small-cell lung cancer on July 30, stage 4. That was six weeks earlier, six weeks carved out of a prognosis of three to six months left to live. At the time of her diagnosis, she was offered chemo, but "my oncologist admitted it was a long, long shot." Instead, she opted to come to Tijuana. "When I asked for a referral to this clinic, my oncologist was really evasive. He said no at first, then said, 'I'll have to read up on it. I'll get back to you.' But he never did."

This was her last day of a two-week treatment. She looked great. "I feel great," she said. "Three weeks ago I thought I was going to die before I even got here. I couldn't walk—I was in a wheelchair because I was so short of breath, I had no strength."

The American Biologics Hospital and Medical Center is an internationally accredited hospital with a full medical staff. It emphasizes an integrative approach to cancer treatment based on the belief that, unlike the conventional interpretation that there are hundreds of kinds of cancer, cancer is one entity with different expressions, the expressions being various tumor types. "Cancer is a chronic, systemic, metabolic dysfunction whose initial cause is at the submicroscopic/genetic level, and of which tumors (including 'tumor types,' 'tissues,' etcetera) are only *symptoms*—however important and at times life-threatening they may be—of the underlying cause. . . . The malignant process itself is our target—not the tissue in which the tumor (or other marker) first was detected. Hence it is our view . . . that cancer (at least epithelially derived cancer) is unitarian in nature; that is, there are not hundreds of kinds and several hundred 'sub-types' of the disease. There is only cancer." (American Biologics, n.d.).

You might be confused right away, because this theory pretty much flies in the face of the descriptions of cancer you hear in the consulting rooms of the cancer clinics back home, that cancer is *not* one disease but many. However, American Biologics agrees with the orthodox world that there is not one magic bullet to cure cancer. "We are not married to any one specific type of therapy. We are not married to any one particular way of doing things," Dr. Rodríguez says, because no two patients are alike, and no two patients will respond the same way to the malignant process let alone to the same general treatment for that process. "We tend to treat everyone in a very individualistic way . . . I feel that there is a place and time for every therapy that we know of."

And this includes some conventional treatments. Along with a range of alternative approaches (Dr. Rodríguez deplores the term, "because it makes you feel that there are only two ways to do medical treatment. One—the conventional way; and the other—the alternative way. I think there is only one and that way is to do it right"), American Biologics uses some chemotherapy drugs, such as cytotoxin, as well as surgery. It also uses the infamous laetrile, or amygdalin, a red flag for conventional practitioners, and the Food and Drug Administration (FDA). "Laetrile is one of the things I would still go for completely," says Rodríguez. "You just have to remember that it doesn't work for every case." The FDA believes that it works in no cases.

Other therapies offered include perfusion hyperthermia (a process of heating the body to kill the cancer cells, which "will self-destruct at forty-two degrees Celsius. Normal cells won't"), EDTA chelation (an intravenous application of a substance to "claw out" toxic heavy metals and minerals from the blood), oxidative and ozone therapies (for "non-surgical diminution of accessible malignant tumors"; bioelectrical therapy ("changes cancer cell polarity and provides an effective, non-surgical, non-toxic approach to one of cancer's major protective mechanisms"); antioxidant therapies (agents to "selectively destroy or inhibit toxic oxygen factors"); nutritional medicine; acupuncture; and B53, which sounds like a bomber aircraft but in fact is genetic material, the lack of which can be the reason for tumor growth.

B53 is manufactured from blood cells. American Biologics gets it from biochemistry laboratories in Seoul, South Korea, but it is also being made in Austria and Germany.

Nutrition is key to many—not all—alternative approaches to cancer therapy: low fat, no preservatives, mostly vegetarian. At American Biologics, it is one of the listed therapies although one of the nurses on the tour was adamant that the orange juice we were served during our presentation was Tang.

American Biologics is both an in-patient and an outpatient facility, treating about 1,200 patients a year. The costs range from US$2,500 for one week of outpatient treatment to $10,000 for the hyperthermia procedure plus $3,900 per week for a three-week stay. A note on the fees schedule says, "These fees are considered to be Deposits against reimbursement by useful [sic] private health insurance programs."

Unfortunately, however, private insurance in the United States is out of financial reach of most Americans. And almost no Medicare/Medicaid insurance will cover American Biologics treatments, although there has been radical progress in the last few years, says Dr. Rodríguez. "I remember the days when I would call an insurance company in the States and I'd say, 'This is Dr. Rodríguez from Tijuana . . . *Click*.' I don't know what has been happening, I don't believe they are just suddenly good-hearted, but this has changed a lot. I would say that 90 percent of the private insurance companies would cover about 80 to 90 percent of treatment here."

Dr. Contreras, the director of the Oasis of Hope Hospital, also in Tijuana, paints a less rosy picture. Later that day he told us that the insurance scene is getting worse, not better; that two years ago, about 70 percent of insurance companies were covering the costs of the treatment at his hospital. Not anymore. But he agreed with Dr. Rodríguez on the adverse impact of the Health Management Organizations (HMOs).

Dr. Rodriguez tried to be tactful about HMOs and gave up. "I hate HMOs. You know because, when you have an ordinary insurance company the boss of the doctor is yourself. You tell the doctor what you like, what you don't like, and if you don't like what he does, you change doctors. Now, in HMOs the boss of the doctor is the HMO. They say, 'Don't treat this patient, don't do X-rays, this patient is too expensive, etcetera.'"

At least one state—Nevada—has brought in legislation protecting patients from HMO practices. This includes laws prohibiting HMOs from offering incentives to doctors for denial of care, and from preventing doctors from telling patients that they have medical options outside their insurance plan. The legislation also states that HMOs must allow medical personnel to help determine the length of hospital stays. In his article "Bitter Medicine," Christopher Hitchens writes, "Every nurse I have spoken to has a personal account of a woman who was sent home, after undergoing a 'drive-through' delivery or breast removal, not on the advice of the hospital staff but on the insistence of an H.M.O." (Hitchens 1998, p. 60). Coverage for alternative cancer therapies is not an option under HMOs.

Canadian health insurance does not cover treatment at any out-of-country alternative therapy centres, and that puts them out of reach for most people.

Like the IAT Clinic in the Bahamas, American Biologics has offered case studies and records of patients for review to the Office of Technical Assessment (OTA) in the United States. To date, the OTA has not followed up on these requests for review, and the treatments continue to be considered "unproven."

The nurses on the tour lace the day with a healthy dose of humor and skepticism. Some are there simply because they need the educational credit. For that they will put up with carrot juice and plates of raw vegetables at lunch and dinner, provided by the clinics. For a while. One woman escapes to a grocery store to buy a Coke, and for a minute she's the most popular woman on the bus. Another complains good-humoredly to a clinic staff member, "This food is bad for my health. Too big a shock to the system. I would kill for a Big Mac." At the next clinic, she nearly gets her wish. Lunch includes a hamburger patty . . . made of tofu.

Our bus finally pulls out of Tijuana's gridlock and squirts onto a fine new highway down the Baja Peninsula. We soar along, the ocean glittering on the right, new construction everywhere, mostly American vacation homes. At Rosarito Beach, the bus bumps along a track that disappears into a washout, creeps up the other side and into the driveway of a building that looks like a great big cottage. The founder of the Santa Monica Hospital, Dr. Kurt Donsbach, says, "I'm not an architect but I designed it based on the fact that I spent nine months as a patient in a hospital at one point in my life and I wanted this to look as little as possible like a hospital." A long, airy building overlooking a magnificent stretch of beach, within hearing of the roaring surf, this hospital is actually welcoming, with its beigey-pink stucco walls, natural woodwork, and signs that say "Please"—"Daily surveys here, please";

"Please leave trays here." The recommended twenty-three-day stay at the sixty-bed facility costs US$15,900, all-inclusive. Companions are encouraged to come with patients—each room has twin beds—at an additional cost of $30 per day for room and board.

The lobby has big squishy recliners grouped around a large-screen television set; the staircase landing is dominated by a huge blow-up photo of the founder standing with President Bush and Barbara. Is this a political statement? Or a message that says, "We're not *that* far out of the mainstream"?

Dr. Donsbach is not only out of the orthodox mainstream, he bucks the current here in Mexico as well. "We have an extraordinarily eclectic way of approaching cancer," he says. "Any way that works I will use . . . until I determine that it doesn't work." (I am immediately reminded of clinical trials—seems to be the same route, smooth for research, pretty bumpy for patients.) "We don't promote any particular therapy over another—we're known for oxygen therapy, but there are so many different oxygen therapies, it is not something that we claim as our own because many people were doing it before we started although perhaps not on the same scale."

What many people aren't doing at the clinics in Mexico is including meat, chicken, fish, and butter in the patients' diet, condemning carrot juice as having too much sugar—"Cancer cells have a voracious appetite for sugar," says Donsbach—or extolling the properties of artificial sweeteners and microwaved food. He is an iconoclast in both worlds.

The hospital's approach is "wholistic," providing a range of therapies including Pulse Modulated Microwave Hyperthermia™; hydrogen peroxide ("Patients drink it, they get it by infusion, they get immersed in it"), ozone therapy, and bovine cartilage. They use bovine rather than shark cartilage because "the effect is better, the science is better and the patients like it better," says

Donsbach. "To be effective with shark cartilage you need 75 grams a day. You feel like a shark, smell like a shark, and taste like a shark with 75 grams. You only need 10 to 12 grams of bovine to get the same effect."

Megadose vitamin therapy is also an important component of cancer treatment at Santa Monica Hospital, an approach that flies directly in the face of the FDA, which is bringing in regulations to restrict vitamin dosages. Donsbach spoke with passion on this subject, obviously infuriated at what he sees as restrictions in the wrong places.

"We use vitamin A here—our average patient gets two million units of vitamin A per day." One of our group asks in disbelief, "Wouldn't that be poisonous?"

Donsbach nods, "Of course it's poisonous. But the patients are all dying anyway. They don't care. And when they live, they realize it's proof that vitamin A is not poisonous. We also use high dosages of vitamin D, which is supposedly toxic also although we never see it. Some of you may have heard how I tried to poison myself with vitamins A and D and took 300,000 units of vitamin A for twenty years and gave up in despair. It seemed I couldn't commit suicide that way."

He grows serious: "One hundred and forty thousand people in the United States alone died of drug overdose last year. I am talking about medicine prescribed by their doctors. How many died of a vitamin overdose? Zero. What are we doing here, folks, this is ridiculous. The FDA has mounted a big campaign, going on right now: they want to put limits on all the vitamins. They want you to have no more than 35 units of vitamin B-6, they want you to have no more than 60 units of vitamin E. Come on, folks. They won't regulate tobacco, they won't regulate booze, they won't regulate a whole bunch of other potentially catastrophic things but they want to regulate nutrition. Why?"

The answer comes back from the floor: "Money?"

Donsbach: "Amen."

Dr. Elizabeth Kaegi, director of medical affairs and cancer control of the National Cancer Institute of Canada and the Canadian Cancer Society from 1993 to 1996, wrote about unconventional cancer therapies for the Task Force on Alternative Therapies of the Canadian Breast Cancer Research Initiative. Megadose vitamin therapy was one. The task force's conclusions were that "There is some laboratory evidence and some clinical evidence that vitamins A, C and E, given separately or in combination, may have value in management of cancer. However, there is lack of solid scientific evidence of the sort required to support a recommendation that cancer patients take vitamin supplements. . . . Further laboratory research is needed to improve our understanding of the functions of vitamins A, C and E and to establish their potential role in the treatment of cancer" (Kaegi 1998 [no. 11], p. 1487).

Hydrazine sulfate is also used at Santa Monica Hospital: "Some of the most noticeable effects from the use of hydrazine sulfate are: increased appetite, mood elevation, increase in strength, decrease in lymph engorgement, feeling of well-being, decrease in tumor size [and] reduction in pain. Because of this extensive research, I have made the decision to use hydrazine sulfate in all cancer cases under therapy at the hospital" (Donsbach and Alsleban 1993, p. 32).

Dr. Kaegi's conclusion on hydrazine sulfate? "Unlike most unconventional therapies, hydrazine sulfate was developed in a way that more closely parallels the development of conventional therapies: a probable mechanism of action was identified and some research using animal models was conducted before the product was made available to patients" (Kaegi 1998 [no. 10], p. 1327). "There is good evidence that hydrazine sulfate inhibits gluconeogenesis. Therefore it *may* play a role in reducing the severity of cachexia and in improving the quality of life of cancer patients. . . . Further clinical research is needed to confirm and quantify the benefits of hydrazine sulfate in reducing the severity of cachexia and improving the quality of life, alone or in combination with conventional chemotherapeutic agents" (ibid., p. 1329).

It appears that there is cautious Canadian support for at least two of the therapies common to most of the Mexican clinics. Very cautious. Too cautious for cancer patients, who don't have time to wait for the further research into therapies that do, right now, make them at least feel better.

When asked about the success or survival rate of his patients, Dr. Donsbach says, "The success rate of chemotherapy is determined by whether or not the tumor shrinks and not whether the patient lives. OK? And if the tumor comes back in three or six months, it's still counted a success. OK? There is a big difference in how we measure our successes compared to how the so-called successes of the allopathic treatments are measured. We did a one-year's study of our patients both here and in our hospital in Poland and found 52 percent of our patients were alive five years later. We did not determine how many of them were free of cancer. But when you consider that this is usually the last stop, when people have been told there is no more hope, go home and die, then they come to Mexico—most of our patients have less than six months to live according to the oncologists—for them to live for five years almost has to mean they are in full remission."

After lunch we clamber back onto the bus and bounce away from the hospital. "When this was built in 1987, there weren't even any roads," the tour guide says. "There still aren't," says a voice from the back of the bus. We head north again to Tijuana and the Meridien Clinic, home of the Gerson therapy, perhaps one of the most famous in the word-of-mouth communications of the alternative therapy world.

The entrance to the clinic is narrow and slightly fortress-like. The initial tone is set by the signs everywhere stating, "Silence is the best medicine." There is a muttering in our group. "If silence is the best medicine, we're in trouble here." "Better than a coffee enema," another answers. We are soon to find out that those signs should indeed have read, "Coffee enemas are the best medicine."

The rather forbidding hallway leads into a beautiful interior garden. Patients' rooms open onto a pool, shade trees, and a profusion of flowers. We are served small containers of carrot and apple juice while Charlotte Gerson, the daughter of the founder of the Gerson therapy, speaks to us. She is a persuasive speaker, charismatic and totally dedicated to her father's theories. All the directors and doctors we heard this whole day spoke of "controlling" cancer. Charlotte Gerson claims to "cure" cancer.

"This is the therapy that almost all alternative therapies are built on," says Gerson. "[It is based] on my father's work in discovering more or less the cause of all chronic diseases, not just cancer—it is the damage caused by toxicity and deficiency that causes the body functions to break down, to be less efficient and causes the immune system to weaken. . . . Cancer is impossible in a normal, healthy, functioning body. So essentially that is what we have to do, we have to restore the normal, healthy, functioning body. And then we see, very interestingly, that it is impossible to heal selectively. When you truly heal the body, all the problems disappear along with the cancer—heart disease, arthritis, high blood pressure, and glaucoma, and on and on and on. True healing means all the body systems are functioning again. And that's the key to the Gerson therapy."

Sounds good, but a little voice nags: too good. *All* problems disappear? I can feel the resistance building to these overarching claims.

"Now, once we understand the underlying problems, that the body's organs are toxic and no longer functioning properly, then it's no longer very difficult to heal. If the underlying problem is toxicity and deficiency, clearly you have to detoxify the patient and flood them with nutrients." Translated, that means juice and enemas. Thirteen glasses of juice a day, and up to five coffee enemas a day. It appears your body becomes a conduit. The daily juice intake provides the body with the nutrients of nearly twenty pounds of organically grown fruit and vegetables a day. Patients also eat generous amounts of raw and cooked solid foods—mostly vegetables—and take thyroid, potassium, and other supplements.

Charlotte Gerson continues: "The juice gets the nutrients into the body. And they go into the damaged tissues and release the toxins . . . into the blood stream and then the blood is filtered by the liver which is supposed to excrete the toxins—if the liver is functional and in good shape." If it isn't, you can further damage the liver. You can get yourself into a liver coma. This is where the coffee enemas come in: "We must help the liver to let go of these accumulated poisons. . . . Caffeine taken rectally has the opposite effect to drinking it. It is absorbed by the colon into the portal system and at the point of the liver it opens these ducts and now the liver can release the accumulated toxins."

Enemas are certainly not a revolutionary new therapy. Archeological finds and papyri, including the Ebers papyrus, dating from about 1550 B.C. and considered the oldest surviving medical book—and the longest, being about 20 metres in length—provide a glimpse of early Egyptian medical practices. The gods governed different body parts, and the physicians dealt in particular diseases or body organs. Physicians were considered healers (along with priests and sorcerers) and, giving new meaning to the expression "royal pain in the ass," boasted such titles as Iri, Keeper of the Royal Rectum, "presumably the pharaoh's enema expert. (Enemas had a divine origin, being invented by the ibis-headed Thoth [god of wisdom])" (Porter 1997a, p. 49).

A patient attending the Meridien Clinic has joined our group for the talk. She sits in the front row nodding her head and emitting little chirps of agreement with every point Gerson makes. Her squeaks get more voluble as the talk progresses. She is turning this presentation into a revival meeting. People around her start to squirm and shoot her looks to silence her enthusiasm. To no avail. She is nearly cheering by the time Gerson finishes speaking.

Dr. Gerson developed his dietary therapy in the 1930s and 1940s and treated hundreds of patients until his death in 1959 at the age of seventy-eight. His daughter has continued his work since. Probably his most famous patient was Dr. Albert Schweitzer whom, according to the clinic brochure, "Gerson cured of advanced diabetes."

The simplicity of the Gerson therapy makes it attractive to many. "There is no scientific mumbo-jumbo to deal with," one tour member told me later. "It is easy to understand. It just makes so much sense." It's simple, but tough. "Not as tough as chemotherapy," one supporter comments. But does it work? The question that was asked at every clinic this day, and answered in a different way by each spokesperson, was put to Ms. Gerson. "The success rate overall is very difficult for me to give you because we have not had a specific study except in one kind of cancer—melanoma—and it's dramatically higher than anything anybody else has shown. In stage 1 and 2 it is 100 percent. For stage 3 it is 73 percent versus orthodox medicine which is 37 percent or so. Stage 4, 38 percent versus orthodox medicine, 6 percent. We're not talking survival. We are talking cure. Because in Dr. Gerson's book, there are three melanoma patients, two are still alive today after forty-five years."

However, at the Centro Hospitalario Internacional Pacifico, S.A. de C.V. (CHIP S.A.), we are told rather petulantly that all the success stats given out by the Meridien Clinic really belong to CHIP S.A. There appears to be a legal tussle over just who owns the real therapy. Or, indeed, what the real therapy is. Charlotte Gerson sticks by the undiluted version handed on by her father. CHIP S.A. has modified it in the form of additional supplements and various therapies aimed at increasing absorption of nutrients.

It was at the Meridien Clinic that other cracks started to appear in the united front presented by the Tijuana clinics. One of our group asked Ms. Gerson what she thought about Dr. Donsbach's claim that carrot juice has too much sugar. Her answer was unequivocal and angry. "But carrot juice doesn't have sugar. I know Santa Monica, and I know Donsbach says, 'Don't give carrot juice.' He is totally wrong. On the other hand, he gives a lot of meat and fish and chicken, and *that's* totally wrong. That feeds the tumor. I would like to see his ten-year-recovered and twenty-year-recovered patients. This is the problem. He does often have immediate results but it doesn't last."

She also disagrees with megavitamin therapy: "Don't take vitamins, especially the oily ones, because you can absolutely cause damage. The tumors grow on the oily ones."

As for vitamin C—she disagrees with guru Linus Pauling as well: "I have a letter in my files from Linus Pauling saying he's not surprised the Gerson therapy works because there is so much vitamin C in the juices, but he is wrong. No one mineral or vitamin can prevent or cure cancer. It's wrong to hang your hat on one thing."

By now, we are a little overwhelmed, and would welcome one thing to hang our hat on. It is the curse of therapeutic approaches to a disease for which there is no certain cure, and no certain knowledge of cause. In the fog of unknowing springs up a welter of choices, mostly contradictory, growing from a rich mix of totally opposing theories. Which are the weeds? Hard to know.

6

The Mexican Tour, Part II

We have three more clinics to visit, and fatigue has taken hold. In some quarters, the resistance is palpable. One of the bus passengers has purchased from the Meridien Clinic a coffee-enema catheter which, as one of the nurses points out, is a urethra catheter. "Maybe they use it because it's smaller," she surmises. "People are giving themselves these enemas at home. Self-inserting a smaller catheter might save on wear and tear." The nurses roar with laughter. Their humor is earthy, their knowledge first-hand and practical, a reality check on the desperate desire for some of the patients to believe every word they hear from the clinic directors, to accept holus-bolus, to sign up on the spot.

The setting sun reflects off the windows of the Oasis of Hope Hospital, an elegant block of marble and glass with a statue in a small garden in the front entrance; two bronze children pick bronze flowers. The hospital is welcoming, with none of the telltale smells of antiseptic and illness. To the right of the main door is the dining area-cum-games room-cum-lounge.

The eclecticism of this hospital is reflected in the odd juxtaposition of the glitzy drum set perched on a raised platform below a huge religious painting of the Good Samaritan offering succor to the sprawled traveler. A large central table is laid out with supper—salads, fruit, and vegetables. It is the Halleluia Buffet, 80 percent raw, 20 percent cooked. No coffee, no tea.

Everyone tucks in except a few of the nurses who have gone into junk-food withdrawal. They rest their heads on their arms, exhausted and hungry for "real food."

Dr. Francesco Contreras, the son of the founder, addresses the group. Tall, well-spoken, and aware that everyone on the tour is tired and overloaded with information, he quickly describes what makes Oasis different from the clinics we have seen. He doesn't say "better," but "different."

"The biggest difference between Oasis and any cancer center around the world is the fact that we are not really worried about what happens to your tumor. You might find that shocking. . . . Orthodox and non-orthodox hospitals focus too much on tumors. . . . They start doing things that are crazy and end up getting rid of the tumors along with the host . . . along with the patient. We believe that what is important to a patient is quality of life for an indefinite period of time. That is the purpose of all of our programs here."

He goes on: "We feel that every injury to the body, every disease to the body, has to do with stress at the emotional level, the spiritual level, and the physical level."

Most of his audience is with him now. Some heads nod in agreement. Stress is absolutely the culprit.

But Arthur and Judy must wonder: what has stress to do with a seven-year-old? How can her body have let her down so quickly. It just doesn't compute.

Dr. Contreras's definition of stress is simple. It is when "your resources are not sufficient to resolve your problems."

The goal of the Oasis staff is to provide you with those resources so that your body can meet the requirements in order to heal itself. Dr. Contreras expands on this: "Unfortunately, in this modern world of medicine, both in the orthodox and the unconventional world, we are boxed into trying to intervene to cure our patients. However, here at Oasis, we believe nobody cures but God."

But this is not faith healing.

Patients at Oasis don't sit back and depend on their faith to cure them. They work at getting better, with the help of therapies and God. "And in most cases God is going to cure you through your immune system," says Dr. Contreras.

Although this mostly means alternative therapies because they provide the resources patients need to help them heal themselves, Oasis is certainly not dogmatic in its attitudes to conventional treatments. Its treatment approach is based on two clear principles:

1. Do no harm.
2. Love your patient as you love yourself.

Within these two criteria, Oasis will consider any treatment, orthodox and alternative, drum rolls and religion. Dr. Contreras makes it clear that any dogma at his hospital is not medical: orthodox treatment is not rejected simply because it is orthodox; nor are alternative treatments to be used simply because they are alternative. This approach partially bridges the gulf between the two worlds.

He gives an example. "If you have cancer that has spread to your liver, your chances of surviving very long are statistically poor. Over our thirty-five years of experience and about fifty thousand patients treated, we know what to expect with our therapies, and about ten years ago our alternative therapies were having the same results as orthodox therapies, that is

0 percent of the [liver cancer] patients were surviving for five years. Very few were surviving for even one year. So we started doing a combination of conventional and unconventional therapies, where we installed a catheter to the liver and we combined laetrile with 5-FU [a chemotherapy]. The liver neutralizes the 5-FU so that very little of it gets to the rest of the body. But the tumor is hit full force by the chemotherapy so you have a lot more of the positive effect and a lot less of the negative effect of chemotherapy. We were able to improve the statistics from 0 percent five-year survival to 30 percent five-year survival. You may say three out of ten is nothing to brag about but it's much better than none out of ten."

Standard therapies at Oasis include detoxification (enemas, colonics, chelation) "because toxins are what are going to be occupying the time of the immune system the most. So if the immune system is going like crazy putting out fires, then it loses its capacity to protect us and that's why we develop diseases," says Contreras.

Diet is important: "We were designed to receive a certain kind of nutrients. So if we provide you with those nutrients, there are fewer toxins for your immune system to deal with."

Immune stimulators are crucial: vitamins, minerals . . . and Jesus Christ. "We respect everybody's beliefs, everybody's religion," he says, "but since we are Christians, we are going to present that view." Prayer is as important as pills.

The Oasis of Hope Hospital is a full research facility sanctioned by the Mexican government. It does no basic research but is allowed to conduct clinical trials on patients provided the products being tested have already been proven non-toxic to humans.

One study now under way is based on the finding that a particular pseudomona is often found in the bodies of people who have died of cancer, suggesting a possible link between the bacterium and the disease. "We have all been looking for years for a link between cancer and bacteria or a fungus or a parasite or any type of bug. . . . Here for the first time is proof that there is one bug constant in patients with cancer no matter what the cancer. . . . It is a pseudomona that has been forgotten for many many years, but we feel that it has a definite effect on the mutation of ordinary cells into cancer cells. . . . the nest for this bug is inside the eyeball."

There are gasps of revulsion from the group. Apparently eye drops have been developed as a treatment that can move into the body systems. "At first we worked with ten patients, all terminal," says Dr. Contreras, "and after seven or eight months, four of ten are still alive. Some have less tumor activity. So statistically speaking we know that this therapy has a big potential."

Oasis is also studying a product from Japan that appears to be a powerful immune-stimulating agent. It has been tested on about thirty patients with all kinds of tumors, both on its own and combined with chemotherapy. Initial results are encouraging. When it was administered to women with advanced breast cancer who were undergoing aggressive chemotherapy in a local hospital, a very high percentage showed no drop in white blood cell count, indicating that it appears to be effective in protecting the bone marrow from chemotherapy degradation.

"The product is derived from a fungus found on the base of very old trees in Japan," Dr. Contreras tells us. "The reason why botanists started studying this fungus was because the trees on which it was growing were extremely healthy in comparison to similar trees in the same area."

One of our group is skeptical: "Oh sure, it's the old rare fungus-among-us therapy," she scoffs.

"You think some chemotherapies aren't weird too?" her table mate answers. "Look at Taxol. It's from the bark of the Pacific yew tree. What's so different?"

Dr. Contreras winds up the question period: "Two more questions and I will let you go on with your tour and you let me go home to my family." It is after 9:30 on a Saturday night.

The two questions were, first, cost—on average, about US$11,000 for a two-week stay plus take-home medication costing between $1,200 and $2,000—and, second, insurance—"About 15 percent of American insurance companies will pay for our treatment, no questions; another 10 to 15 percent will pay after a lot of work. We are trying to hook up with a company from Florida. . . . " But he's not very hopeful: "Since the whole HMO scandal in the United States, the insurance is a lot tougher."

The Oasis presentation finishes with a tour of the hospital. The young man who had introduced Dr. Contreras leads us along the hallway almost at a gallop, gesturing at closed doors: this is our lab, this is our surgical room, this is our laundry, down there is administration. He hurries us along, scooping up a security guard to unlock an empty room to show us the accommodation for patients and their companions.

When asked a medical question, the young man said with such honesty you had to like him, "I'm not a doctor, you know. I'm just the PR guy."

Genesis West, the second last clinic on our itinerary, could have done with a PR guy. We trailed off the bus, up a dark path, and into a large, dimly lit room. Out of the twilight, a row of dentist chairs took shape; you could just make out the trays of picks, drills, and probes—the standard-issue tools of the trade for your average Spanish Inquisitor—at the head of each.

The gloom, the glinting instruments, and the occasional flash of reflected light off the Coke-bottle eyeglasses of our greeter transported us into a bad Hollywood horror flick. One nurse spun on her heel and hurried back to the bus; Judy quietly escaped onto the terrace and took pictures of the small, leaf-strewn pool, greenly glowing in the dark. Someone behind me started humming the theme song to *The Twilight Zone*, and stopped abruptly when the greeter began to speak. It was the director, Dr. Swilling. Ramrod straight, with a frozen smile, he welcomed us, and with his first words, the presence of the dentist chairs was explained. "Causal factors are used to guide the treatment for each and every person. We have found with that focus that many of the cancers and other degenerative diseases have their origin in the mouth."

In the pause following this statement you could hear jaws clenching all over the room. Dr. Swilling explained that the culprits lurking in our mouths are not just amalgams which leak heavy-metal toxins into our systems, but also root canals. "We have discovered that most breast cancers can be traced directly to infections in root canals. It has to do with acupuncture points. The infection sets up an inflammatory path to mammary glands and causes tumors. When we remove the root canals, the tumors become benign. The first thing we do here is check the patient's mouth for mercury fillings and root canals. Only when they are replaced can we proceed with treatment."

In other words, the teeth would have to be pulled before treatment would start.

But once you get past the teeth thing, many of the treatments offered at Genesis West are similar to those of the other clinics, although the theory upon which they are based appears to differ somewhat.

Dr. Swilling says, with no false modesty, "In my twenty years as a research scientist in the field of biochemistry and chemical nutrition, I have been able to understand and comprehend the nature of disease." Disease is a multi-causal problem. The trouble starts when the body gets out of balance. His theory is that when the body's pH level gets out of balance and becomes too alkaline, then it can't absorb nutrients from food and so attacks itself for those nutrients. It turns from anabolic to what Swilling calls "catabolic."

Minerals are essential in maintaining the proper level of pH. When there is no assimilation of minerals, the metabolic functions of the cells slow down, and the resulting fermentation in the cell consumes so much oxygen that the cell becomes anaerobic. The lower the level of oxygen, the more likely the complete breakdown of the cellular system. "This is the nature of the degenerative process," says Dr. Swilling. That slowdown is associated with disease, and leads to the development of cancer.

As simple as that. To the layperson, this is not simple. To an exhausted layperson, brimful with claims, counter-claims, theories, and admonitions, it might as well be Greek, a form of chemical doublespeak that effectively extinguishes even the most determined attempt at understanding.

To restore the balance, Genesis works with nutrition: forms of minerals distilled from sea water, hydrochloric acid mixed in special foods and drinks.

Ozone therapy administered directly into the vein with dimethyl sulfoxide (DMSO), auto-haemotherapies to oxygenate the blood, rectal insufflations, vaginal insufflations, aerobic baths—all these apparently help to detoxify and evaporate the fermentation in the cell.

Dr. Swilling is openly critical of the medical establishment. "It has become my mission," he says, "not only to work one on one with a patient in the clinic situation but to bring this information to people who are seeking how to take charge of their own health in the face of a failing medical system that is actually creating more illness and disease than any other factor in our lifestyles."

He finishes his presentation with the statement, "I hope we will be making contact with you guys in the future."

"I don't think so," mutters the woman standing beside me. "I absolutely don't think so."

But back on the bus, another passenger leans over the back of the seat to talk. She's convinced that Dr. Swilling is right. "You know, I got breast cancer two years ago. And I'd had a root canal the year before." She had heard of this theory before visiting Genesis West, and had already had one root-canal procedure removed. She was saving up to have the second one done.

The folks at the Centro Hospitalario Internacional Pacifico, S.A. de C.V. (CHIP S.A., pronounced *shipsa*) patiently waited for us to turn up; we were now three hours late. Dr. Ron Carreño acknowledged our long day and promised to make his presentation short. He did. Not by taking anything out but by talking very, very fast. He fired his words in a shrapnel stream of data—like tracer bullets, the medical bytes fly over most of our heads. He is utterly devoted to his subject, committed to the therapy and to the founder of CHIP S.A., Dr. Issels. And he expects that same commitment from his patients:

"When I see people come into this hospital . . . and if I see they are not going to keep things up, I will stand up, I will close my book, and I will refer them to another hospital . . . ."

The CHIP S.A. approach begins with an immunology review including blood chemistry, heavy-metal testing of the urine, a full physical examination and—wait for it—"evaluation of the teeth and tonsils for root canals, dead or devitalized teeth, leaking mercury amalgams, impacted wisdom teeth, incompatible amalgams, periodontal disease, hypertrophic, atrophic and septic tonsils" (CHIP S.A. information sheet).

Dr. Ron, as his colleagues and patients call him, describes Dr. Issels as "the father of modern biological dentistry." So important is it to get the immune system working properly that "in this hospital, you had three days to have your teeth and tonsils taken care of—otherwise you were asked to leave. It wasn't open for discussion. It was not because Dr. Issels was being mean, it was because he wanted to help you out—he cared so much. . . . he couldn't be in the presence of someone who didn't care."

Dr. Issels died in February 1998. It is not clear whether patients are still given only three days to have their mouths sorted out. When asked the question, Dr. Carreño simply reasserted the need to do so. The information sheet says, "If immune system is frozen, jolt with immune modulators, remove root canals, dead teeth, impacted wisdom teeth, leaking amalgam teeth, problem tonsils, incompatible tonsils." It doesn't say incompatible with what.

From the "rock bottom base of good nutrition" (the Gerson diet) and detoxification, CHIP S.A.'s treatments—called "immune system stimulating factors"—can include chelation; natural interferon producers (Tagamet, L-carnitine, melatonin); high-dose vitamins; Coley's toxins; shark cartilage; ultraviolet blood irradiation; hyperthermia treatments; vaccines; and hyperbaric oxygen treatment. Also listed among the medical procedures are "laughter, exercise and lots of prayer."

"When you start on [our] therapy," Dr. Ron tells us, "you become like a fine-tuned engine. The juices are one part, the enemas are another part, but this is a full program. There is the nutrition base, and then detoxification, but all the medications we give are to try to increase the absorption. It doesn't do you any good if we give you all the nutrition but you can't absorb it."

He uses a metaphor to explain: "All the additives we are giving are based on the fact that God gave us this wonderful organism and it has the capability to spring back. If you take an old car, put some new gas in it, put some air in the tires, do a tune-up on it, the thing starts running. Case in point: you saw an old car in the parking lot when you came in, a Nissan Sentra; that's my car, and it's still running. That's based on the same system."

Is this good science? Not really, but it's well-received comic relief, a life raft in a sea of complicated descriptions of metabolics, COQ10, ATP changing to ADP, immune-profile testing of CD3, CD4, CD8. . . . Heads are drooping again.

After a rapid-fire talk by Mrs. Issels, the wife of the founder, Dr. Ron came back with slides of various patients. Because of the late hour, he snicked through them at a rate of knots, so that the tumors on these people appeared to melt away like wax. The testimonials offered by the clinics and hospitals are always slightly suspect because they have an agenda. But these were impressive, especially the ones showing the efficacy of hyperbaric oxygen treatments on the healing process. One slide showed a sad-looking man with an enormous tumor down his face and neck, and apparently in both lungs. He was known as "the sourpuss." He stayed in his room, did not smile. He could not smile, for godsake. Successive slides showed a smaller and smaller tumor. Then Dr. Ron called to someone in the back, and "John, the sourpuss" walked up to the front of the room, no tumor in evidence, a big smile in place.

I was not the only person in the group uneasy with this form of exhibiting the success of a therapy. It brought to mind . . . circuses.

But John spoke simply and movingly, not so much about his own case, but about how difficult it is to make decisions. "I wouldn't presume to tell you what to do, but try and use logic—don't let price or emotion get to you. Think it all through and try and find a logical solution for yourself. The most important decision is whether you are going for conventional therapy or alternative therapy. I would urge you to go for alternative therapy first, because conventional therapy is so damaging. If all else fails you can go backward."

One of the tour guides hit the gong to indicate we absolutely had to go. A quick tour of the hospital and then we were back to the bus, followed closely by Dr. Ron and Mrs. Issels, still talking, their fervor genuine but overwhelming.

Our final stop, Manner Clinic, got short shrift because it came at the end of an exhausting day. We filed into the lobby and the director began his presentation immediately, sensing a rising tide of sleep among his audience.

"When a patient comes to this clinic they say, 'I have one problem,' but we have to look at all the problems to find out why they developed the disease. We find out that they eat junk food for example. . . . " *Quelle horreur.* Not *junk food.*

A thin, high voice rose from our midst: "I *love* junk food, I *want* junk food." And it went downhill from there. The tour of the clinic was a shambles. We wandered in and out of rooms, lost the tour guides, and were eventually rounded up and steered into an upstairs dining room. There were cookies and juice and a quick talk by three of the staff before we shuffled out again.

The clinic is named after Dr. Harold W. Manner who was its director from 1982 until his death in 1988. Born and raised in New York, Dr. Manner received his M.S. and Ph.D. from Northwestern University before launching an illustrious university teaching and research career, including appointments as chair of the biology departments at Syracuse University, St. Louis University, and finally at Loyola University in Chicago. He retired in 1982 to devote himself full time to his work in metabolic therapies. He edged into confrontation with the establishment over laetrile, the therapy that ignited a raging controversy throughout medical circles in the 1970s and 1980s. "Few controversies in cancer therapy have been as fierce or prolonged as that over the proposed anticancer agent laetrile." Its detractors call it "goddamned quackery," its proponents hail it as "one of the most promising and effective treatments for cancer" (Moss 1996, p. 131). And, as always, desperate cancer patients are stretched on the rack between the two camps.

Laetrile is no newcomer either in our diets or in medical use. Apparently Peking Man ate it (in the form of fruit kernels), and it was used as a preparation "useful against tumors" as early as the first or second century A.D. in China. Its presence is like pepper throughout the soup of medical history: Ancient Egyptian, Greek, Roman, and Arabic physicians used versions of it, and "Celsus, Scribonius Largus, Galen, Pliny the Elder, Marcellus Empiricus, and Avicenna all used preparations containing laetrile to treat tumors" (ibid., p. 133).

Such lineage must be one of the longest in medical history, but that doesn't necessarily mean that laetrile works. It does mean that it should not automatically be cast into the shadow of quackery, dismissed contemptuously as at best useless, at worst poisonous. Its detractors like to point out that it is cyanide. Its defenders counter by listing all the other "cyanides" we eat every day—chick peas, lentils, barley, brown rice, cashews, and the ubiquitous lima beans. Laetrile occurs naturally in about 1,200 different plants around the world.

The word *laetrile* coined by Ernst Krebs, Sr., in 1953, refers to a purified form of amygdalin, a substance first isolated in 1830 from bitter almonds. He, and his son Ernst Krebs, Jr., registered the term and patented their purification method, but the small-l laetrile usually refers to the various commercial forms of amygdalin currently used in cancer treatment today (ibid., p. 133).

Some believe that the laetrile controversy is much more than a dispute over a single agent in cancer treatment. "Laetrile and the movement that has grown up around it pose a major challenge to the current methods of treating cancer as they are practiced at most medical centers. This challenge has not only medical but also philosophical and socioeconomic implications. Laetrilists are not just advocating a single substance but, like the advocates of other unorthodox therapies, are proposing a new kind of treatment for the patient's body and mind" (ibid., p. 134). This was the theme that gave resonance to all the therapies we heard about on the Mexican clinic tour: cancer can be controlled (in some cases the claim is "cancer can be cured") through the enhancement of the body's natural defenses—the immune system—rather than through methods that attempt to destroy it directly.

When Dr. Manner moved to Loyola University, he wanted to orient the work of his department toward Lake Michigan. Among other things, "Research funding would probably come easier because the federal government was at that time concerned about water pollution" (Manner 1989, p. 1). It is ironic that a journey that started with an attempt to ingratiate himself with the federal authorities ended in a conflict that drove him from his university and his country. His research into carcinogenic properties of water pollution led him first to the laetrile theory. "I laughed when I read this theory because it appeared to me to be an extreme oversimplification of an answer to what I then felt was a highly sophisticated and complicated disease. Basically the theory stated that the extract of an apricot kernel—Laetrile or Vitamin B-17—when taken into the body, circulated around the blood stream until it met a cancer cell. At the site of the cancer cell, an enzyme, produced by the cancer cell, triggered the release of a deadly compound, called hydrocyanic acid (HCN). This cyanide compound killed the cancer cells" (ibid., p. 3).

The theory stayed with Manner (it "gnawed at my insides") until finally he called his research group together and suggested that they test the theory in a laboratory setting. It was at this point that he discovered he was walking into a war, not a scientific debate. "Instead of finding sound scientific dialogue in the available literature, we found charges and counter charges . . . not based on scientific data. . . . Political pressure and legality or pseudo-legality raised their ugly heads. . . . Offers to meet in parked cars and in out-of-the-way coffee shops were very numerous" (ibid., pp. 3–4).

Dr. Manner was the first scientist to conduct large-scale animal studies using laetrile with a combination of vitamins, minerals, and enzymes. The results were startlingly positive but "greeted with skepticism by most cancer researchers" (Moss 1996, p. 145). Manner was criticized for presenting his findings to a lay group first, for not testing the various elements separately, and for not publishing in scientific journals. "The establishment had much to say against Manner but, as the Chicago scientist often pointed out, orthodox cancer research doctors never availed themselves of the opportunity to refute his claims *by refuting his tests*" (ibid., p. 146, emphasis in original).

I had expected to hear much more about laetrile on this tour—the facilities in Tijuana are often referred to as the laetrile clinics—but in the presentations it was not often singled out as more than one of many complementary treatment approaches. At the Oasis of Hope Hospital, Dr. Contreras, whose father was a major player in the early laetrile wars, said: "Just about all our patients receive laetrile because we have proof over many many years that laetrile has a mild but sure antitumor effect."

When asked about its legality in the United States, he said, "It is definitely not FDA approved, that I can tell you. For sure, though, if you are a patient who comes to Mexico for treatment you can legally take your medication back home and a doctor can legally give it to you. You can also order a three months' supply every time and legally use it for your own malignancy. You cannot share it or sell it."

Dr. Ian Mackay, head of the Special Access Program of the Health Protection Branch of Health Canada, says that for the most part, laetrile has been dismissed as "not having potential" in fighting cancer. However, theoretically a physician could obtain it for a patient under the program.

The laetrile controversy continues, although less hysterically than twenty years ago when the FDA posted "Laetrile Warning" posters in 10,000 post offices across the United States. It is legal in twenty-seven states but there are few manufacturers of the substance within the country. Since it is illegal to transport it across state borders, it is difficult to come by. And the total polarization of beliefs exists to this day. A ten-minute Internet search in October 1999 turned up these diametrically opposed opinions on laetrile:

The Laetrile phenomenon started with a pharmacist-physician who developed one concoction after another for the treatment of serious diseases, especially cancer. It continued with his son, a self-imagined scientist, who spent many years in college but failed to earn any graduate degree. A man who earned his fortune from gun-running and a Catholic newspaper columnist promoted it as a persecuted drug that cured cancer. A cadre of John Birch Society members saw the repression of Laetrile as a sinister plot against their basic freedoms. After it was dubbed "vitamin B-17," an army of health food devotees promoted Laetrile, along with vitamins and diet, as nature's answer to cancer. . . . After peaking in the late 1970s, the "Laetrile Movement" ran out of steam . . . as the Laetrile fantasy faded, its prime movers added many other "miracle cures" to their arsenal and added AIDS, arthritis, cardiovascular disease, and multiple sclerosis to the list of diseases they claim to treat. Although they appear to speak with sincerity, they still fail to sponsor the type of research which could persuade the scientific world that anything they offer is effective (Wilson 1999, no page numbers).

But:

During 1950 after many years of research, a dedicated biochemist by the name of Dr. Ernst T. Krebs isolated a new vitamin that he numbered B17 and called "Laetrile." As the years rolled by, thousands became convinced that Krebs had finally found the complete control for all cancers, a conviction that even more people share today. Back in 1950 Ernst Krebs could have had little idea of the hornet's nest he was about to stir up. The pharmaceutical multinationals, unable to patent or claim exclusive rights to the vitamin, launched a propaganda attack of unprecedented viciousness against B17, despite the fact that hard proof of its efficiency in controlling all forms of cancer surrounds us in overwhelming abundance. (Vialls 1999, no page numbers)

Our tour was over. It was midnight and the bus was quiet. A few reading lights shone in the darkness. As we neared the border, our guide gave us instructions: take everything with you when you get off the bus, don't offer any information, stick together as you walk through the customs and immigration shed. The bus will be searched and then pick you up on the other side of the border. In case we had picked up any aliens.

As we filed past the immigration officers, we were each asked, "What nationality? Where were you born?"

"American. The United States."

"American. The United States."

"Canadian. Canada." I was waved out of the line.

"Identification?" Then: "What did you acquire in Mexico? Just the usual tourist crap?"

I nodded numbly. Easier to go with the lie. He waved me through to the land of the free.

As we waited for our bus again, a fellow passenger said, "I am so totally confused. I would hate to have to make a decision right now on which therapy to choose."

"I *do* have to make a decision. By Wednesday. That's when I'm due to start radiation," said another. After he retired, he was diagnosed with prostate cancer. He had surgery. "They took my prostate and the only sphincter that was any use. My doctor said, 'I'm sorry, I thought I got it all, but I didn't.'" The cancer had already spread. "Now I have carcinoma of the rear."

"Rear??" I repeated in disbelief.

"Ear. Ear." He slapped the side of his head. "They don't seem to know if it's the same cancer or a new one. I've got to tell my doctor tomorrow that I'm not taking his treatment. I feel bad, he's a nice guy. He got me in for radiation quickly. But I'm not doing it." He paused, then said to no one in particular, to the world, "Anyone tells you about the golden years? Don't believe 'em. It's a pile of crap."

He picked up his bulging shopping bag of literature and videos collected from all the clinics and climbed back on the bus. Judy and Art were the last two to get back on. In their exhaustion, they looked so alike, vulnerable, sad. Art now faced the toughest decision he will ever make.

The difficulty of choosing is not unique to the alternative therapy world but it is made tougher there by the lack of professional review and the clandestine atmosphere of the search. Because of the establishment's stranglehold on cancer treatment, and its hostility to alternative therapies, patients must rely on their own judgment, their own visceral responses to the various therapies. And on top of this they are made to feel guilty for looking beyond the conventional for treatment. A foray into Tijuana's seedy byways is reminiscent of the bad old days of searching for a backstreet abortionist. There was an unease among some of the passengers on that bus, papered over with jokes and bravado; many wondered out loud how they had arrived here in their lives, traveling with strangers in a foreign land, forced to search beyond the borders of their country, beyond the borders of the cancer wards back home, not just for access to the treatments themselves but for access to *information* about them.

Patients looking for options within the conventional parameters have easier information channels to follow, signposted by practitioners yoked by their common belief in the relatively narrow mainstream approaches. And usually they don't have to search alone or with strangers, without the support of their original doctors. Rarely must they conduct site visits of the Mayo Clinic, say, or Toronto's Princess Margaret Hospital to help decide on a treatment. If they did, they would probably be as bewildered as many of the people on the Tijuana tour.

The need for such a tour rises from the "closed shop" attitude of the cancer establishment, and it is a bizarre experience for cancer patients searching for another way. After about the third clinic, a sense of unreality started to take hold. Here we were, a bus full of very disparate, many desperate, souls on a grotesque shopping tour—but cancer treatments are not discount drugs. A bus tour is not a firm foundation for good choices. But what are the options? The medical establishment paints the alternative world with the brush of sleaze and fraud. The Cancer Control Society's bus tour tries to give people the opportunity of direct observation, however superficial, of this world. The theory is that then they can decide for themselves, without having to filter out the censure of those whose opinions are based on second-hand information. But to have to make a crucial decision on treatment choices based on a bus tour of seven or eight clinics in a day is a mockery, a sad commentary on a medical system that puts individuals into such a position.

7

Surviving Against All Odds

Growing public interest in alternative medicine is a worrisome development for many practitioners of conventional medicine, particularly in cancer treatment. Their biggest objection is that alternative approaches draw people away from mainstream methods they feel have a proven track record. Some people ask, track record for what? For beating cancer? No. For controlling cancer? Sometimes. And there's the rub. Increasing numbers of cancer patients would not be tempted to leave a treatment if it weren't so destructive and if they knew it was going to work.

"The use of cancer treatment without proved benefit has become a major public health issue, with substantial numbers of patients deserting potentially curative conventional therapy in favour of unproved methods. . . . As patients and the public have become increasingly educated, dissatisfaction with conventional cancer care has grown. The toxic effects of chemotherapy, the absence of new and markedly improved treatments despite decades of effort, and the lack of substantive improvement in rates of cure for the major cancers all contribute to the dissatisfaction" (Cassileth 1991, p. 1180).

Some people "desert" mainstream approaches because they've exhausted what is there for them. They are making a choice, not between therapies, but to continue to fight the disease on another medical front. The unconventional therapy is their last resort. Their risk could be seen as less than those who make unconventional therapy their first choice, the ones who look at the statistical odds, or at other patients ravaged by therapy as well as disease, and flee at the beginning of treatment.

It is a huge decision, to abandon the ship of conventional cancer therapy for whatever reason and at whatever point in the journey. What kind of person makes the jump? What event, what sort of attitude, pushes an individual over the side?

Lena Bos was diagnosed with breast cancer in 1986. That started her on a twelve-year odyssey in search of a treatment that would halt the disease raging in her body. Lena has had every treatment conventional medicine could provide and, when they didn't work, she turned to alternatives, clandestine clinics within the United States, non-conventional centers outside the country—fever-bath treatments in Alabama, electromagnetic treatments in Tennessee, laetrile treatments in Tijuana, and finally immuno-augmentative therapy in the Bahamas.

Lena's journey began with surgery. The surgeon who performed the radical mastectomy said that he'd got all the cancer. She was home free, no need for any other treatment. According to some benchmarks she really was "cured" at that time because she was cancer-free for four and a half years. Try telling Lena that. Approximately every year since 1990, the cancer has come back, first in the other breast, then on the chest wall, then in the lung, and finally in the bones. More surgery, then chemotherapy, then radiation, then more chemotherapy, and more radiation—but the cancer kept coming back.

Enough, already. Lena opted for a bone-marrow transplant or, more accurately, "peripheral stem cell harvest and transfusion." Her doctor told her that 99 percent of patients are cured by this procedure. "Those that survive the treatment," her husband, Elmer, adds. This it how it went:

Lena and Elmer go to New York. "We checked into the hospital," Lena says. This is not the royal "we." It was during these visits that Elmer earned his reputation as the husband who wouldn't go home: "The nurse told me to go to my motel, that they had no facilities for overnight visitors, but I didn't care. I was happy to sit in a chair by Lena's bed. They pretty soon arranged for a mattress for me."

Lena was hooked up to a machine and for ten days, three hours a day, her stem cells were extracted until they had enough to see her through what was coming next. She and Elmer went home to Grand Rapids, Michigan, and Lena had three months of "aggressive" chemotherapy. "This is where they throw the book at you," says Elmer. This is where doctors are forced to put aside their very first promise—"To do no harm." Then back to New York for more chemo, this time by continuous intravenous for about thirty hours. After three days' recovery time, Lena went back into the hospital where she was given back about a third of her stem cells. Then home.

In ten days Lena was so sick she spent the next two weeks in hospital getting blood transfusions. They barely hung on to her. But she was strong, she recovered. And went through the same procedure two more times. She nearly died, they iced down a fever gone out of control, she was delirious. She had no hair, no eyelashes; she was skin and bones, and she fought back. Now, the cancer must be gone, because her doctor did say 99 percent of patients do not get cancer back after a bone-marrow transplant. Lena grew stronger, put on some weight; her hair grew back. One year later, so did her cancer. She was the 1 percent.

Her doctor appeared to have exaggerated the odds somewhat. Perhaps that's the bookie's prerogative, to adjust the percentages according to the context. A review from Seattle of 3,635 patients showed that 865 developed complications needing mechanical ventilation for more than twenty-four hours, and only fifty-three patients survived (*Annals of Internal Medicine* 1996). However you play with the stats here, it does not add up to 99 percent survival.

This time Lena had a tumor in the lung. No problem, her surgeon said. We'll just go in and nip it out. "Just going in" meant through her back, breaking ribs on the way. One IAT patient who had had the operation describes it from the point of view of the "operatee": "It is brutal, they break you across the table like an egg—flip open your ribs and have a good poke around." Lena still has pain from this surgery. They mopped up any residual cancer with Taxol, a very toxic chemotherapy. Away went her strength, her weight, her hair. But not her spirit. And not her cancer.

Lena heals very quickly. She has to, to allow time for the next invasion. A year later, a tumor appeared in the lung again. Her doctor prescribed more chemotherapy. When Lena said, "NO," he was surprised: "Why not?" He didn't seem to have been paying much attention—chemo had not worked for Lena. But cancer was still not through with her. She developed pain in her hip. X-rays and a bone scan weren't conclusive. Elmer wanted her to have radiation, but the doctor said, "We can't radiate unless we're sure of what we've got here." "With her history?" Elmer asked in disbelief.

When the tumor was big enough—because what they'd got there was indeed cancer—Lena had radiation. Then the pain started in her other hip. Pretty soon Lena could not walk because of the pain. Again her doctor downplayed its seriousness but finally agreed to do an X-ray. He phoned the next day: "Is Lena sitting down?" Actually, she couldn't do much else. "Because she mustn't walk or her leg might break. Tumor has eaten away the femur."

More surgery. A pin was put into her leg from hip to knee, followed by more radiation. While the bone was healing, another tumor appeared just above the old site.

That was when Lena started to look at alternative therapies, unable to withstand the ravages of the frontal attack of conventional treatment any longer. "They weren't helping anymore, and I couldn't just sit at home and wait to die."

Marcia Frank chose another route to IAT—the direct one. Diagnosed with breast cancer in November 1996, Marcia had a mastectomy, and cancer was found in twenty-seven lymph nodes.

"It doesn't much matter after ten," Marcia says. "Early detection? Oh, puleeese. Don't talk to me about early detection. I've been mammographied, palpated, and poked nearly to death over the last five years, and this lump did not show up. I kept going back, saying I think there is something wrong, it hurts, it feels funny. When the nipple inverted and the breast started puckering, they said that a biopsy was needed. The diagnosis was lobular carcinoma which, they pointed out, sometimes does not show up in a mammogram. Now they tell me!"

Marcia's mother had breast cancer, a mastectomy, and cobalt treatments that left Marcia with a searing physical image of the disease—or at least its treatment. The radiation therapy had left her mother's flesh blackened, raw, and suppurating. "I was not going to have breast cancer," Marcia smiles ruefully. "I am a vegetarian, I did yoga, meditated, laughed, I had joy—but always I had fear. It was always in the back of my mind—I will not be my mother."

After her surgery, Marcia was advised to take high-dose chemotherapy followed by radiation. She said, "I know that's not going to work for me." Her oncologist called her at home, "You must come and do this treatment. Without it you have a 90 percent chance of recurrence." With it? Seventy percent chance of recurrence. "I could not do it," Marcia says.

When she told her son and daughter, both in their thirties, they tried to persuade their mother to "do the right thing," to change her mind. Her husband, Peter, supported her decision, but was anguished. "To know where to go is so difficult."

Marcia knew, though. "I try to listen to my instincts—to my heart. That's how I found [IAT]—by following my heart."

Like Marcia, Paul Schubert chose the alternative route at the beginning of his journey.

Paul is tanned, his body lean and fit from an active lifestyle. He looks the picture of health. Paul has Dukes D stage-4 colon cancer. A routine blood test in December 1996—part of the annual physical checkup required by his company—indicated that he was anaemic. A retest confirmed that something was indeed wrong. CAT scans and a colonoscopy revealed a five-centimeter tumor and lesions on and in the liver. How had they been missed before? Could the cancer have developed within a year? Not likely. As Paul says, "We all had a lot of faith in the medical profession, but they can't catch everything."

His prognosis was not good. "The way it works, the lower down the alphabet the worse it is. D is worse then B." Paul says ruefully, "I don't think it goes lower than D."

His wife, Fran, asked the doctor, "Do you not think he is going to make it? I mean what are his chances?" "He just shook his head. He just shook his head for a while and said, 'They are not good. Not when it's gone this far and it is in the liver.'"

Paul says, "My wife—she's a real fighter—and my brothers were in the recovery room after my surgery and they basically said, 'We're here and we are going to create a battle plan for how to fight this thing.' I had told Fran, before they found out for sure that it was cancer, 'Worst-case scenario: if this is cancer I don't want chemotherapy.' I have seen too many people, known too many people, who have done chemotherapy and their quality of life is just terrible. They're so sick and it just seems like all they do is go downhill."

They researched everything they could, alternative, traditional, everything, to give Paul the information he needed to decide what to do. "It is his life and he had to make the decision, so we wanted to be very careful not to steer him one way or another," Fran says. "But I wanted him to get a really clear picture that he was not by any means a done deal. He had a whole lot of life and fighting to do."

The surgeon introduced them to an oncologist who told them what he thought their options were. "Let me ask you a question," Paul said to him. "You've been in practice for a number of years, you have treated a lot of patients with the same thing that I have. How many of them have you cured with chemotherapy?" If "cure" is defined as five years without recurrence, the answer was "one."

Paul said then, " 'So what you're telling me is that I have a very slim chance that chemo would have any effect on me.' He said that it would buy me a couple more years maybe. . . . But Fran had talked to the National Cancer Institute plus the National Institutes of Health and got several studies, protocols from them about new treatments, possible experimental things. . . . One of the studies was of the exact same cancer and stage that I have, treated with the same chemotherapy the oncologist wanted to use on me. Their study came flat out and said there was no evidence that chemo extended life at all. At the most maybe two months. And this is from the National Cancer Institute. So here is the oncologist telling me that chemotherapy could buy me another couple of years, and the study from totally the top institute in the country for cancer research is saying that with my level of cancer there is no evidence that it does anything for you. When I think about this, I get really angry. They are treating thousands and thousands of patients and they know that it doesn't work. So we put together our battle plan." A plan that brought them to the IAT Clinic in the Bahamas.

"You know, those people who have come down here, they are not really thumbing their noses, but they do not do what traditional medicine wants them to do; they are taking a big risk," Fran says. "I think it takes a very special kind of personality to have the strength to do that. I admire them so much."

Paul says nothing for a moment and then speaks quietly. "First of all, death doesn't scare me. When I think about it I worry about Fran and my family and how much I love them and the life I have with them. But what's beyond, I am not afraid of that. What I am afraid of is not being able to live my life to the fullest extent, whatever length of time that might be. So it wasn't courage, maybe fear because I didn't want to take something that I knew would make me sick and diminish the time I have left. And it is still hard to accept the fact that I have cancer, because I feel so good."

Right? Wrong? All these people made choices. They chose to "desert" the system to take control of their own lives and health. Is this so radical, when a doctor says, "There is nothing we can do for you," or "We can try this new experimental chemotherapy, it might buy you a month or two."

A spirit of survival is at work here. All these people have taken control against serious odds.

This spirit is not unique to those mavericks who seek therapies beyond the conventional. You see it in patients everywhere, the ones who are going to "beat" this disease. "Beating cancer" doesn't necessarily mean living for ever, or at least dying of something else at the end of a long life. It can mean, for some, living until next Sunday, for others, extending a prognosis of six months to six years. It means, for these people who have made such difficult choices, not dying before dying. These are the survivors.

Dwight is a farmer/sailor with melanoma, "the queen of cancers, because it can go anywhere," he says. It has. He has eight tumors in the groin.

"My surgeon said to me: 'You have five options—none of them will work.'" Dwight had come to IAT on a trial basis. "Dr. C. told me, 'We don't have much success with your kind of cancer: only 25 percent of similar patients have had extended life and good quality.' Well 25 percent is about 24 percent better than my surgeon offered with his five conventional treatments."

Dwight went on, "You wanna see dead? Go to the malls in Florida—these old geezers died years ago and they're still walking the malls. I'm sixty-two years old, I've lived full, I am living full. I'll be living right up to when I'm dead, not the other way around, not dying up to when I'm dead."

Dwight said this at dinner one night and very nearly got a standing ovation. A group of IAT patients and their spouses, friends, and partners had gathered at Buccaneer's Cove, a restaurant a few miles from Freeport. A few of the patients were leaving the next day; a few had just returned for their tune-up. Good enough excuse for a party.

Steve Gibbons was one of the patients about to leave, anxious to get home to his family, his work, his life . . . well . . . his *other* life. Because life certainly hadn't stopped here for him.

When Steve first arrived at IAT, he was suspicious, scared, almost willing the therapy not to work. Another patient described him with great affection as, "the no-alternative-therapy-for-me Steve." Steve worked in the insurance business, a world of blue, cold statistics and arctic actuarial realities where long shots don't belong.

When Steve's second surgery revealed a host of further tumors in his colon, chemo was now apparently the only option left. He had his first treatment a month after surgery, at about the same time a client of his told him about the IAT Clinic. "I wasn't too interested, because chemo seemed to be working. I did phone my client's cousin who was a patient at IAT. I was told that he was in the Bahamas for a tune-up. Whatever that meant."

Steve didn't pursue it. That was in April.

By November, his oncologist told him the chemo was no longer working. Steve relates the conversation.

"What do I do now?"

"Well, we have another chemical, CPT-11. Sloan-Kettering says that with this new drug they have been having 'significant success with the prolongation of life.' Quote, unquote."

"How long?"

"I don't really know. It differs with each patient."

It turned out that the "prolongation of life" meant anywhere from three to eleven months. And the side effects were vicious: nausea, hair loss, mental confusion, loss of balance. ...

"This was life?" Steve demands with indignation. "More like 'life sentence.' If there was a chance of real surviving I would have taken it, but for the sick miserable months offered, it wasn't an option. I'd rather live a few months well, and then die. Not live a few sick months and then die anyway."

The oncologist told Steve's wife, "There's nothing more we can do then, except pain control."

Steve called the IAT patient again. "Not here. He's in the Bahamas for a tune-up."

"Jeez, does the guy *live* down there?"

His client was in his office a few days later. "Did you call my cousin yet?" Steve told him he was in the Bahamas.

The client, "who had an arm like a thigh," slammed his fist on Steve's desk and roared, "What the hell is wrong with you? God dammit, you think they don't have phones in the Bahamas?"

Steve called the Bahamas and talked to Jerry, who had been coming to IAT for seven years, with the same cancer and metastasis as Steve. Here was the option.

"You have nothing to lose," Jerry told Steve. "In two to four weeks, they'll send you home if you're not responding." Steve was not sent home in two weeks. Now, looking fit and healthy, and full of energy, he was going home after eleven weeks. "Jerry had described how great the place was, the ambiance, the patients, the staff. But you know, he'd understated the camaraderie, the lack of stress. I arrived here tired and apprehensive, and the pain had already started. But I got right with the flow. I've never had so much freedom in my life, never felt better."

Another dinner party, this time at Coral Beach, a small apartment hotel on the ocean near Port Lucaya, outside Freeport. Seçkin and Dave (he has liver cancer), Diane (lung cancer), and Annabel (mesothelioma) all arrive with identical thermal freezer bags slung from their shoulders. Diane plans to sew some Christmas glitter on her serum bag for next week's parties. She's going home for Christmas—home being Montreal. She puts two bottles of wine on the table . . . and beeps. Time for a needle. Timers go off all night. At one point, a beep sounds, and everyone looks at each other, "That's yours, isn't it?" "Nope, not mine, must be yours." A kind of gruesome version of cell-phone society was at play here. The answer to the imperative of those beeps and rings was self-inflicted needle jabs, not a "Let's do lunch" conversation.

Seçkin and David Wieting are from Turkey, where he was diagnosed with liver cancer that seems to have developed from hepatitis C. They don't know how long he has had the cancer. Dave says, "In 1973, everything was fine; in 1980, apparently I had slightly elevated liver function," but only recently had he developed any symptoms. The swelling in his feet and ankles was first diagnosed as rheumatoid arthritis. But when the swelling was not reduced by medication, further tests were ordered.

His oncologist in Turkey told him that he had less than a year. "With chemo you might get an extra year, but at what cost? You must decide between quality and quantity."

David opted for quality.

Diane Loader had her lung cancer diagnosis confirmed over the phone. Until that phone call, after all the weeks of tests, and the assurance that her symptoms were caused by hypertension, no one had said the word "cancer." Her oncologist now told her that with this form of lung cancer there was no treatment, and it was not a matter of years but of months.

When she asked him if he thought she should consider an alternative therapy, he said no, "Unless you want to waste your money, then go for it." His "alternative therapy," Diane says, "was 'Wait until you are sick and then we'll give you chemo,'" as palliative treatment. "When I asked about a support group, he suggested I see a psychiatrist."

Diane's lung specialist also said that they had no treatment to offer but that he had a patient who had gone to IAT and had done very well. She translated her own pathology reports from French to English and sent them to the clinic with a covering note: "If I don't hear from you by Friday night, I will be on your doorstep Thursday morning." This letter, in her file, has the notation on it "OK to accept, 8 Nov. 96."

Diane is matter of fact about the sudden changes in her life: "I only found out the weekend before [arriving at the IAT Clinic] that I had to give myself shots every day. It hadn't really dawned on me. I thought, well, OK, OK. My father-in-law is a diabetic so he has been giving himself insulin shots all those years and I thought that was terrible, but I don't think so anymore."

Diane stayed in Freeport until February (with a week home for Christmas), and on her return to Montreal went back to her lung specialist. When he saw her new X-rays, Diane says, "He couldn't believe it. The tumors had not disappeared but they had not grown either. 'We couldn't have done this,' he told me. 'This is unbelievable. If you were doing chemo, we'd say it was working.'"

In June, it was the same story. She went back to IAT for her two-week tune-up, returned to Montreal, and had more tests. Her specialist brought in interns this time, "'Can you believe this?' he asked them, and said to me, 'I don't know what they are doing but you keep doing it.'"

Annabel Brown, from Toronto, has mesothelioma, a cancer that incubates over years and, by the time it is diagnosed, usually kills within months. Since her arrival at the clinic, she looks a little better, though she is still very pale and her "beer stomach," as she calls it, is still very extended. X-rays are showing nothing abnormal. She is only slightly reassured. She is quiet, but when she does speak it is with a strong clear voice.

Dave, on the other hand, might as well be speaking from the bottom of the sea. Seçkin says, "What am I going to do with this little man of mine? He is losing his voice."

"This little man" who towers over her, grates out cheerfully, "I am being consumed." The image is instant—a malignant mass inching up from his liver into his throat. Again, the jauntiness. None of this is self-delusion. They all appear to have faced the beast, recognizing that there is a good chance it will devour them; but they seem to have come to some kind of quiet resolution to fight like hell, all the while watching themselves from the sidelines. It is an odd thing—you see that attitude in some patients, not in others.

Seçkin starts to tell anecdotes. "This is not just a Turkish story," she says, making quotation marks with her hands. "This is FACT." She laughs.

"The oncologist in Turkey said Dave was to have chemo. We said no. He said, 'This is inoperable,' and showed us the X-rays. A large tumor in each lobe of the liver, with small ones in between. We went to the United States, and the oncologist there said much the same thing, but there was a surgeon at Sloan-Kettering. He got in touch, the surgeon said yes, he could operate."

Wait a minute, how was that possible? The doctor in Turkey said it was inoperable. Whom to believe? So they contacted another doctor at Sloan-Kettering, a woman oncologist. Her advice? Indeed, her warning? "Don't come here, this is a research hospital."

It appeared that Dave was in such dire straits that the doctors saw him as a guinea pig. "It would be good for medical science." Seçkin rolls her eyes in disbelief.

Dave, although his body is still distended with fluid and riddled with cancer, is eating well, feeling better. Diane looks fabulous, glowing with excitement about going home for Christmas, feeling great. Annabel, for the first time since leaving Toronto, is without pain. She is content, quiet, enjoying the conversation, at ease for the moment, feeling better.

Lena Bos says, "When I came here first I couldn't do anything, I was depressed, couldn't read, could barely lift a hand. But now my energy is coming back, I feel stronger. . . . I walked two blocks this morning. I haven't done that for a long time."

Steve has "never felt better" after eleven weeks of treatment.

OK, feeling better is good. But are they *getting* better? Not necessarily the same thing, as so many critics point out in the discussion about the relationship between attitudes—the mind—and a patient's health—the body. This debate, which has raged for centuries, bristles with issues. Holistic practices have swung in and out of favor, suffering a body blow with the ascendancy of "scientific medicine," but enjoying a return to favor with the burgeoning interest in many forms of alternative therapies. It is interesting to note here that while Hippocrates has been adopted as the father of modern (i.e., scientific) medicine, another group of medicants who lived at the same time as Hippocrates were the forerunners of medical practices that much more closely resemble the conventional medical practices of today. "It is one of the ironies of this history [of medicine] that the academy of Cos, the so-called Coan school [Hippocrates' crowd], had a rival, situated on the opposite peninsula at Cnidus. . . . The Cnidian focus was on the disease, while that of Hippocrates was on the patient. The Cnidian physicians, like those of today, were reductionists, fine-tuners who directed their efforts to the classification of the processes of sickness and to exact diagnosis" (Nuland 1995, pp. 8–9).

In the last decade there have been several studies of the impact of attitudes and emotions on an individual's ability to cope with or recover from illness. As usual, they arrive at conflicting conclusions.

A Stanford University study of breast cancer patients published in 1989 showed that women who participated in a support group lived thirty-six months longer—twice as long—as women in the control group who received the same medical care but without the support services (Drum 1998, p. 195).

A study of AIDS patients measuring the immune system's response to support groups that focused on coping and relaxing skills found that the patients' immune systems were actually stimulated, as shown by their higher levels of natural killer (NK) white blood cells as compared to those of patients not in support groups (ibid., pp. 195–96).

A Dartmouth Medical School study found that heart patients were fourteen times more likely to die following surgery if they did not participate in group activities and did not find comfort and support in a religious belief.

In a randomized, controlled trial of eighty-six women with metastatic breast cancer, fifty were assigned to weekly supportive group therapy and were taught self-hypnosis for pain control. The other thirty-six women were not. The entire group received conventional treatment. Follow-up showed that the women in the support group lived an average of 36.6 months after the trial began, compared to the controls (the women who had only straight medical treatment), who lived an average of 18.9 months (Fugh-Berman 1999a).

On the other hand, a 1993 study comparing advanced breast cancer patients who attended Dr. Bernie Siegal's support group sessions for what he calls Exceptional Cancer Patients

(ECaP) and patients who received the same medical services but did not attend the support group meetings found no difference in survival rates between the two groups (Buckman 1996, p. 346).

So the jury is out on whether mental attitudes can prolong life. But what about the quality of the life left. One of Dr. Buckman's patients sums it up beautifully: "Even if feeling better is not the same as getting better, isn't feeling better a whole lot better than feeling worse?" (ibid., p. 336).

Most patients would agree. Why would you submit to a therapy that at best will buy a few months of miserable life rather than a few months of quality life? Bill Britton's searing description of his wife's experience in a chemotherapy ward in Scotland sums it up:

> The difference between my wife here [at the IAT Clinic in the Bahamas] and in the hospital [in Scotland] is that she believed that the therapy was going to do her some good and certainly that it was not going to do her any harm. In the hospital, even though it was a friend who was administering the chemotherapy, we could see the lady on the left [in the treatment room] had a great big fat neck from the chemotherapy; the lady in the center bed was going blind . . . from the chemotherapy. The lady on the right was going deaf . . . from chemotherapy. And the lady next to her had a kind of a stroke . . . from chemotherapy. We began to realize that chemotherapy does more damage than I think we understand. So this is something you realize; if you are not going to suffer, have no bad effects and live on a beautiful island like this, and [you have a chance] to get better as well . . .

One of the conclusions of the Cassileth study comparing survival and quality of life among patients taking conventional and non-conventional treatment is that treatment and its side effects alone do not determine quality of life. The response to this finding from most cancer patients is, "No kidding. You need a study to find that out?" But such studies are the only tickets to acceptance in the world where credibility rests only on science.

8

When the Fighting Stops, Can We Start the War?

That's the scene then: conventional and alternative therapies nose to nose, both worlds laced with issues that reach out and snare cancer patients just trying to get healthy. Even if you keep your head down, your eyes firmly fixed on the narrow trail in front of you, you can't avoid the players, the debates, and the questions.

First of all, most practitioners of conventional cancer treatment come down like gangbusters on those who espouse any method that isn't. And vice versa. Cancer patients caught in the middle ask themselves why there is such vitriol, why the two sides sit poles apart.

The usual spawning ground for prejudice is generalization, stereotyping, forcing a whole range of similar but different elements into a box where they become an easy target for thoughtless attack. That is what happens here. Within the broad category of non-conventional/unconventional/ alternative therapies fall a host of approaches, some barely recognizable as being relatives. Immunotherapy is lumped in with shark cartilage, which is painted with the same brush as coffee enemas, which are yoked with Chinese herbal medicine. The fact that some approaches might work better with one form of cancer and not with another seems to be overlooked in the rush to condemn them all.

The confrontation may come partly from alternative cancer practitioners' paranoia and frustration at being frozen out by the medical establishment. Some, too, might fear exposure of fraudulent methods.

It may also come partly from conventional doctors' fear that they risk their entire professional career by entertaining anything beyond the scope of their training. "I've studied for ten years to be a good doctor; I'm not going to be shunted aside by someone who learned his craft from his grandmother who learned it from her grandmother. Knowing how to collect and mix herbs is going to cure cancer? Rubbish. Clinical trials are the only way to establish the efficacy of treatments. The cure can only be in a test tube at the end of decades of meticulous trial-and-error research."

But many alternative therapists *are* researchers; they have used the scientific method from the beginning—first studying, then working within the confines of science (Burton is one example). The big divergence is the clinical-trial stage—testing the drugs or therapies on humans, the stage at which new treatments are tested against old ones, or against placebos. There are many doctors who object to this practice, not only alternative practitioners. Theirs is not necessarily a shifty-eyed sidestepping of the final test, but a genuine worry about ethics.

Fear of change is a great motivator for pulling up the drawbridge against anything new. "New" equals "suspect." It threatens the dogma of the establishment, whether in religion, in medicine, or in law. But often in the world of medicine today's heresies are tomorrow's cures. Look at its history. In the 1840s, for example, obstetrician Ignaz Semmelweis worked out the cause of childbed fever, which was killing up to 25 percent of mothers after childbirth. At the time, most physicians thought it was either a specific disease, like smallpox, which came and went as an epidemic, or a miasma floating in the air from some noxious source. Semmelweis discovered that it was a transmittable but not contagious disease, and stoppable through the simple expedient of having doctors wash their hands in a chlorine solution between patients. Unfortunately, he was before his time. He presented a disease concept the medical world wasn't ready for. His theory was based on the idea of bacterial contamination nine years before Louis Pasteur discovered bacteria and more than a quarter of a century before Lister proved that infections were caused by bacteria. His simple rule of hygiene, which a few years later was to become a cardinal rule in medical practice, was rejected. Obstetricians continued for years to go from one delivery to the next without washing their hands or instruments, killing their patients in the process. Rejection of the new or different is a powerful retardant of progress.

The history of cancer treatment provides a context to the current medical disagreements. Our twentieth-century skirmishes are depressingly familiar, depressing because for 2,500 years we appear to have been fighting versions of the same battles again and again; real progress seems to be in spite of, rather than because of, these debates. No one wins them; they just reappear in slightly different guises throughout medical history. For instance, "In the second century, theories of disease causation were still based, as they would be for centuries to come, upon the Coan factors of climate, diet, geographical location, occupation, temperament, and the effects of each on the balance of the four humors" (Nuland 1995, p. 40).

The scientific method scotched these theories, replacing the big picture with the minuscule by proclaiming the presence of germs, viruses, bacilli, and everything else that squirmed under the scientific microscope of observation and studies. This was progress, no question, but on one level those second-century theories hold sway again. We are coming full circle with the growing evidence of the impact of environmental factors—"climate, diet, geographical location, occupation"—on incidence of disease. The "temperament" of that quote resonates with the current personality theories of disease: the Type A personality that incubates heart disease, Type B that does not, and Type C, the repressive, self-effacing disposition that breeds cancers.

And this: in the second century, "[t]herapies were somewhat more aggressive than they had been five centuries earlier, though there is no evidence that they were any more successful, and a large number of botanical and animal products had entered upon the therapeutic scene, which seem to have been prescribed with an enthusiasm that was not justified by any demonstration of their efficacy" (Nuland 1955, p. 40). Replace "botanical and animal products" with "chemotherapy" and you have just transferred that observation from the second to the twentieth century without losing a jot of accuracy.

On your Pilgrim's Progress from cancer diagnosis through a variety of approaches and treatments, you will also encounter a variety of players, good, bad, and indifferent. What makes it even more confusing is that the Good Guys are not all on the same side.

The dramatis personae on the medical stage include:

- Doctors trained within the establishment who cling, blinkered, to their training, rejecting anything from outside the fold—the conservatives.

- Doctors trained within the establishment who are open to new ideas and new approaches, spurred on by the failure of the conventional approaches to stop cancer—the moderates.

- Doctors trained within the establishment who reject their training and embrace new therapies, again driven by failure of the traditional methods and frustrated by the snail's pace of development of sanctioned therapies—the mavericks.

- Scientists and researchers with strong medical background who work painstakingly, moving in tiny increments of progress. They come in two forms—the workhorses and the thoroughbreds.

- Scientists and researchers, scorned for not being medical doctors (though they never claimed to be) but with strong scientific and research skills, who develop a medical therapy from a base other than traditional medical training—the innovators.

- Entrepreneurs who exploit the market, attracted by the lure of the Big Buck (not averse to helping people, but only as a secondary goal)—the carpetbaggers.

- CEOs and leaders of big business conglomerates/government organizations whose barely hidden bottom line is profits (while they claim that their activities are solely for the common good)—the hypocrites.

- Hucksters and out-and-out deceivers who are in it for the money (and perhaps personal power), who deceive and trick and connive—the criminals.

Faced with all these players and their competing agendas, you might simply decide to back away from it all and take control of your own treatment decisions, turning inward and to other cancer patients for help and guidance. Support groups in the last few years have proliferated. In Toronto,

Willow Breast Cancer Support and Resource Service for women with breast cancer, is the hub of a network of more than sixty-four groups in Ontario alone. Because of market demand (a trendy way of saying that breast cancer won't go away), a galaxy of breast cancer organizations exist, encompassing advocacy, information, support, funding, and rage that there is still such denial in high places of the links between environmental toxins and what is now being called an epidemic, and such resistance to doing anything about it. These groups are founded, organized, and kept going mostly by "survivors," women with breast cancer whose spirit is large enough to fight both the private war with their own disease and a public war to change the status quo. In the face of the daunting mortality rate in such groups, the spirit of survival flourishes against considerable odds.

"Taking control" is a phrase often heard now in the cancer world. Patients are becoming their own case managers because so often no one else is doing it for them. They are having to coordinate their own care, and in doing so they must make decisions based on conflicting information from warring medical experts. Some would argue that this situation is healthy and liberating. We are given the risk factors for a disease; we are told that prevention is the answer—which often translates into a simplistic prescription to keep cancer at bay through lifestyle choices. But with the freedom—or necessity—of choice, comes responsibility, and with responsibility often comes guilt.

So not only do you have the players to sort out, you have the issues that trail the treatment approaches to this disease. Do you *want* to be able to choose your own route? Do you have the information to make sensible choices? *Are* there sensible choices? What do you do when you read of yet another breakthrough which, under scrutiny, turns to dust? What do you do when medical science tells you that you are at high risk for getting cancer and in the same breath says that there is nothing yet you can do about it? How do you know when a recommendation to go into a clinical trial is really for your benefit, or just for the benefit of science? What do you do when clinical trials of the same drug arrive at conflicting results?

Or, you might wonder, do you even have the right to choose? Will the authorities step in and squelch your freedom of choice if you go too far afield? You might ask, are they doing this honestly for the good of my health, or is the motivating force something less honorable? You hear often about the cancer "industry"—are protectionist forces at work here because of economic or social imperatives?

Bill and Kathy O'Neill tumbled into this teeming world of questions the summer their son Liam developed headaches. Their story is a microcosm of all the Big Ticket issues a patient deals with in cancer care, and the turf wars that still disfigure the landscape. The horror of their experience was heightened by the fact that it was their child who was threatened.

The summer of 1992 promised to be a good one. Weather forecasts called for warm temperatures, lots of sun, and enough rain to keep the farmers happy. It was mid-June, and all the kids in the land were poised to burst from their schools, heads buzzing with plans for the long, hot days ahead. Roll on summer, bike hikes and basketball, hammock days and long splashy swims, late-day treks to McDonald's, the Dairy Queen, the Burger King, and all the ice-cream places with outside tables and moths diving into the lights at dusk and darkness. The O'Neills had family plans for a camping trip, a road trip and a whole month at their cottage in West Quebec.

Bill O'Neill was a computer analyst for the City of Ottawa, Kathy worked in early-childhood education. They had three kids—Kelly, fourteen, sociable and starting to pull away into her own teen world; Liam, twelve, shy, creative and on the threshold of a summer of promise that included passionate involvement in all that he did; and Gareth, eight, following Liam's lead, but already carving his own way. Liam was his best friend, and Gareth would follow him anywhere. That summer, Liam went somewhere that no one could follow.

Nothing went according to plan that summer. It turned out to be one of the wettest and coldest on record. And the O'Neills' August and September slowly darkened as clouds of another sort gathered over their lives.

Liam's headaches were occasional at first, then more frequent and more severe. They heralded the beginnings of an odyssey that would take him to the brink of death, change his family's lives forever, and launch his parents on new careers.

By the end of September, Liam's headaches are hitting him every two days. No longer just a pounding sensation after physical exertion and a tightness, now the pain is much worse. Bill and Kathy take him repeatedly to their family doctor, and they just as repeatedly get the same reassurance. There is nothing to get upset about. Lots of kids get migraines. Or perhaps he has a food allergy. Or they could be growing pains. "In his head?" Bill asks incredulously. Liam's headaches persist and worsen. So do the visits to the doctor, who grows impatient. She tells Bill that he is overreacting when he insists on tests and referral to some sort of specialist, a neurologist, a cardiovascular specialist, an endocrinologist, anyone who would help. Finally, the doctor agrees to send Liam for blood tests. Liam collapses and has a seizure right there in the lab. Bill and Kathy are frantic. The GP is inexplicably nonchalant. No connection to the headaches, she says, but agrees that Liam should see a specialist.

When the neurosurgeon examines Liam, he does not prevaricate: "This boy has a brain tumor." No ifs, buts, or delays to the diagnosis. Liam is rushed to the hospital for a CT scan and a craniectomy and has surgery within two days. The tumor is malignant.

That is how it began: a parents' worst nightmare, watching their child suffer, and as it turns out, at least some of the suffering needless. A rite of passage for Liam that most children never have to experience—pain, frustration, fear, and the shocking realization that the "authorities" in the adult world are fallible. Indeed, more than fallible, culpable.

Liam is initially diagnosed as stage 1 medulloblastoma. The hospital recommends radiation treatment. Staging tests are conducted: bone marrow—negative; cerebral spinal fluid—negative; myelogram (X-ray of the spinal cord)—positive. According to the radiologist, the film indicates a tumor in the spine. Metastasis. The cancer has already spread. Liam is now stage 4 medulloblastoma, which means he needs chemotherapy as well—"relapse/salvage chemotherapy," Bill says. "They kept telling us, 'Maybe he'll have two good years, but it [the cancer] always comes back.'"

The radiation treatments really take it out of him. The surgical site becomes red and swollen, but when Bill and Kathy ask if it could be an infection they are assured not, that it is cellulitis from the radiation. Liam needs blood transfusions; he sleeps all the time. His decline is blamed on the naturopathic and homeopathic supplements his parents are giving him.

"We were in and out of the oncology clinic three or four times a week," Bill says. "And we were reminded over and over again just how bad Liam's prognosis was." When Bill continues to question, challenge, and offer information from his own extensive research, he is referred to a psychiatrist because he is "in denial."

The surgery wound is looking angrier and angrier, and Bill and Kathy worry that if it is an infection, surely chemotherapy should not be started. "Liam had his first hit," Bill says. "Two days infused chemo." Five days later blood tests indicate that his white blood cell count is practically zero—his immune system has been wiped out. "We were told to watch for fever," Bill recounts. "He has a fever. They [the oncology physicians] want to see him. He's readmitted at Emergency and placed into protective isolation. They're still saying he does not have an infection at the surgery site."

Kathy and Bill are beside themselves. Their world has fallen apart. Kathy keeps a journal, writes poetry to keep herself sane. So does Liam.

Kathy writes:

Irish Superstitions
The father asks,
"What does it mean when a picture falls?"
And spends hours repairing the frame.
"If I can fix this, he'll be fine."
Cleaning his room,
Clothes and toys left where he dropped them.
Another poster slowly slides down the wall.
Pounding it into place the mother screams,
"You can't have him yet!"

Liam writes:

> tall
> skinny
>
> a grinning
> bald
> panicked boy
>
> sitting
> eating
> spoonfuls
> of sugar
>
> wondering why
> he's so
> hyper

The site on Liam's head erupts. The oncology team now acknowledges infection. When the surgeon, who has been out of the loop on Liam's follow-up care after the operation, hears what has happened, he's furious, wants to know when the infection started, why he wasn't told, who was involved. The infection gets worse and Liam is in isolation for nearly a month before he is allowed home.

The oncologist continues to press for the next chemotherapy treatment. "Neurology and Infectious Diseases were saying no to chemo," Bill says, "and in the meantime the oncologist says to Liam—remember this is a twelve-year-old kid—'I think we should do another CT scan to make sure there aren't any more tumors growing in there.'"

On February 16, 1993, an MRI study is done of Liam's head and spine. MRI (magnetic resonance imaging) is a highly sophisticated technique that produces internal pictures of the body using electromagnets, radio frequency waves, and a computer. "MRI appears to be the most effective procedure for diagnosis of head and neck cancers. Investigation of the neurological system (brain and spinal cord) is best accomplished by MRI" (Altman and Sarg 1992, p. 182).

"We waited in anticipation for the results," says Bill, "even though the radiologist told us it would be too soon to see any changes in the spinal mass." Apparently the radiologist was wrong. The oncologist tells Bill and Kathy that the spinal mass is gone. "We were ecstatic. We thought that would mean no more chemo for Liam. But she told us that wasn't the case and reminded us again that with stage 4, the cancer always comes back."

On April 13, at the regular cancer clinic visit, Kathy and Bill are waiting to consult with the doctor in the examination room. Liam's chart and records are there too. Kathy finds a radiology report of the MRI conducted on February 16 which indicates, as the oncologist reported, that there is no spinal mass. "It also says there *never* had been a spinal mass," Bill says. "The results of the myelogram had been pulled again, and the report confirmed that it had been misread."

"Finally we get it. Liam has been misdiagnosed. We raised the report with the resident oncologist who agreed. Liam is stage 1 not 4. He should not be getting chemotherapy."

Liam's odyssey began with the horror of the diagnosis of cancer; it was made more hellish by the misreading of a test result which led to treatment that nearly killed him; but the nightmare did not end with the discovery of the mistake, because, according to Liam's parents, it was compounded by a denial, a cover-up, and the team oncologist's insistence on proceeding with more chemotherapy even after the inaccurate staging of the cancer was revealed.

Relations between the presiding oncologist and Liam's parents grow more than frosty; they become almost non-existent. "When I met with her [after Kathy's discovery]," says Bill, "she was still convinced that Liam had metastasis to the spine and had to have more chemo. She was cross about the letter in the file, not because of what it said, but because it was left in with Liam's records."

Bill and Kathy ask that Liam's records and test results be sent to the Montreal Neurological Institute (MNI) and St. Jude Children's Research Hospital in Memphis for second opinions. The oncologist agrees. They are to meet again in a week. Bill phones the two hospitals to confirm that they have Liam's records. "They've never heard from Dr. X, and don't know who the hell Liam O'Neill is. Yet she insisted that she had made the referrals to the people I had just talked to. Those referrals never did happen. Then we asked for referral and possible transfer to Sick Kids (the Hospital for Sick Children) in Toronto. She agreed to send everything down— charts, film, everything. A week before we go, I call Sick Kids. No charts, no film, nothing. I call the [oncologist], she's not available. The receptionist says that the charts and film will be sent that day. I called the next day and was told that the oncologist was sending a letter but no charts and film. I asked to speak to her directly but she wouldn't talk to me. So I spoke to my lawyer."

When Liam's records finally made their way to Toronto, the O'Neills received confirmation that Liam's brain tumor was stage 1, not stage 4.

Liam is now a healthy, normal kid who survived the disease, the treatment, and a medical system gone awry. He's no longer the "bald panicked boy," although he still has the same puckish sense of humor. But he has been forever changed by his experience, not just with the disease but with his treatment and the way it was handled.

The facts of this story and the events that propel the "plot" sound like fiction: the misread X-ray, the administration of unnecessary chemotherapy, the letter in Liam's medical file that led to his parents' discovery of the mistake; conflicts between the attending specialists; the circling of the medical wagons to protect their own; a lawsuit; the total disruption of life for Liam and his family; the launching of a new career first for Bill and then for Kathy; and finally, at the end, a remarkable boy who, with the help of determined and unintimidated parents, has survived it all.

The broader implications of this story touch so many of the issues patients find themselves struggling with after a diagnosis of cancer. Trying to get information, for instance. During Liam's trial by error and terror, Bill missed so much time at work that he lost his job. Not a problem. His new career had already sprung from Liam's experience, fertilized by rage at the information dead ends and the doublespeak of the medical team treating his son. Through every step of Liam's treatment, Bill and Kathy asked questions. At first they were polite, they deferred to the doctors' wisdom. Then their questions became more insistent, more probing, more challenging. Finally, they stopped asking questions, and went searching for answers elsewhere. In 1993 Bill launched his new company, the Canadian Cancer Research Group (CCRG), to help patients punch through those dead ends that he and Kathy had encountered onto the information highway of knowledge and choices worldwide. It was a timely move. The Internet was exploding, and medical databases were proliferating. It was an information jungle; Bill was the guide, digging out facts specifically relevant to his clients' situation.

After a couple of years, more information providers appeared, and people also became more adept at ferreting out data on their own. But by then the O'Neills had already made the move away from information provision, first to providing access to alternative cancer treatments, and latterly to providing the treatments directly through the CCRG.

Most oncologists are wary of Bill O'Neill and his group, labeling him Dr. Hype. But patients who are on some of the treatments provided by CCRG call him Dr. Hope. He's not a doctor, although one oncologist flatly refused to believe this, asking him to consult on some cancer cases. His medical team now includes GPs, pharmacologists, and biochemists. No oncologists, though, because (he grins slyly), "Most oncologists are not qualified to treat cancer."

"It's like this," he says.

Artificially built constructs prop up conventional cancer care, and they are perpetuated by media and medicine that have this institutionalized myopia. It's like, we can't look at anything outside our box, outside our training. The plain and simple fact of the matter is that [oncologists] don't have one clue, because if they did, they would be doing it [successfully treating cancer], but they don't have a clue. . . . When you take on the vested interests you are called controversial. How can I be called controversial— because I help people? No, it's because I'm challenging the status quo.

He believes that there is a renaissance happening, brought on by a growing resistance to a society that is being destroyed by powerful, manipulative forces:

We have been blindsided by industry and medicine since World War II: we are being sold things that don't work, or that hurt us; the environment is totally fucked; the incidence of cancer is rising; but people now want to make sense of things, to determine if something is based on good sense, in science, in medicine, in industry, or whatever. Do chemo and radiotherapy make sense? Absolutely not. Cancer is not the bald-headed kid. That's the treatment. Cancer is such a horrible disease. Well, no. We have a bunch of incompetent systems run by incompetent myopic people who have completely fabricated a sociological and clinical standard, not on the basis of the disease and our ability to manage it but simply on our failure and unwillingness to consider any different paradigms in medicine and thought.

Bill does not choose his words carefully. His son's experience has effectively deleted any diplomacy; he is a very angry man, and is content to antagonize the medical establishment he believes nearly killed his boy.

9

Freedom of Choice: Licence or Liberty?

The freedom of medical choice: just whose is it? The government's or the individual's? Karen was on the Mexican bus tour of alternative cancer centers because she had run out of options; her breast cancer had metastasized to her lungs and liver. A bone scan scheduled for later that week would likely confirm that the pain in her hip was also cancer. The man with prostate cancer was on the tour because he wasn't willing to submit to any more radiation and chemotherapy, treatments that he felt had depersonalized him to the extent that he was nothing more than his disease. Judy and Art were there in search of a less destructive treatment for Art's seven-year-old daughter, already reeling from her first belt of chemo. And one passenger was there because she was frightened of the lack of options in the United States. "I don't have cancer . . . yet," she said. "But I'll know what to do when I get it." She was already preparing her route in the new world of cancer therapy because she didn't like the main highways that were the only choice back home.

Paul Schubert left a hospital in the United States after surgery for metastatic colon cancer and went to the IAT Clinic for a treatment he believed in, turning away from one that he didn't, and the only one that was offered back home. Diane Loader left Montreal for the IAT Clinic because her doctors said they had nothing to offer except a prognosis measured in months, not years. Lena Bos abandoned conventional treatment only after years of chemotherapy and radiation culminating in an unsuccessful bone-marrow transplant at Johns Hopkins. She tried fever-bath treatments and electromagnetic treatments at clandestine clinics operating in Tennessee and Alabama; she went to Oasis in Tijuana, and then to the IAT Clinic.

Liam O'Neill has never been back to the hospital where his treatment for a mis-staged brain tumor brought him near death. His father, Bill, now brings in alternative treatments not previously available in Canada, transporting theories and therapies here rather than sending the patients across borders. Tyrell Dueck, the thirteen-year-old boy with osteosarcoma who fled his Canadian oncologists and surgeons, was released from the imperative of conventional treatment only by evidence that his disease had spread to his lungs. The courts had ruled that he must undergo more chemotherapy and have his leg amputated on the evidence presented by his doctors that this approach had a 70 percent chance of curing him. There are many who dispute this statistic, but not the courts. It was enough to take the control of his treatment away from Tyrell and his parents, who were charged with failing to provide the necessities of life. "But in Tyrell's case the judge failed to ask the doctors for proof supporting their opinion. . . . With other professions they seek evidence," Bill O'Neill says. "Why is it that even our courts abdicate to these people [doctors] as if they reside higher in the food chain."

Dr. Sue Aitken, from Ottawa, was also outraged at this decision: "As an oncologist, I know how fast sarcomas can move. What those doctors and the court put this boy and his family through was unconscionable, absolutely wrong."

The people on the Mexican tour, the people at IAT, and Tyrell are only a few of a growing population trying to establish their right to medical treatment of their own choice in defiance of the decrees of those "stern protector[s] of the most rigorous brand of science," the federal regulators and conventional practitioners in their own countries. Because their decision has taken them beyond the borders of conventional medicine, they have had, in most cases, to cross geographical borders as well. So cancer isn't the only thing they have in common. Their medical odyssey has turned them into exiles, and in the eyes of their own governments they are taking part in illegal practices, decreed so in the name of their own protection.

Many cancer patients suggest it is ironic that they must leave the lands of the free to exercise their medical freedom of choice. The other side of the argument is that such agencies as the U.S. Food and Drug Administration, the Health Protection Branch of Health Canada and the provincial colleges of surgeons and physicians are protecting citizens from fraud and misadventure—and themselves. It is a thorny issue. Certainly, not all alternatives are benign. A bad choice can lead to a quicker death, as was the case in the horrific story aired on CBC's *Market Place* in January 1999. Stasha Roman was dying of inflammatory breast cancer, a lethal, fast-growing form of the disease. After surgery, chemo, and radiation failed to stem it, she and her family went to Mexico on the advice of a health food store owner in Manitoba. The "clinic"—the Vallarta Rejuvenation Center in Puerto Vallarta—wasn't a clinic at all, but a house with barely adequate cooking facilities and even less adequate medical arrangements. The doctor in attendance visited only every other day. The man who ran the clinic claimed to be a doctor of naturopathy, but in Mexico to practice naturopathy you must be registered with the Ministry of Health. He wasn't. One of Ms. Roman's treatments was to be wrapped in a plastic bag and have ozone blown over her. At one point, her husband reported, there was no proper bag so she was wrapped in a plastic sheet taped closed around her. For this the family paid $19,000, and she died within ten days of returning to Canada. There are many similar stories of people who fall into the hands of hucksters.

The regulatory agencies and authorities are charged with protecting patients from just such occurrences. They have rules in place to protect the public good, to encourage progress in medical science along replicable lines, and to eliminate quacks and nutters. One of the ways they do this is by imposing rigid requirements for bringing all cancer therapies through from initial research and development to the marketplace. Plastic bags with ozone would not get through the starting gate.

But despite the good reasons for these requirements, the process is unwieldy, slow, and expensive, well beyond the reach of individual researchers or small labs. Critics point out that the system is geared now to large pharmaceutical companies, the only ones able to afford it.

These agencies are criticized when they fail to protect the public as, for example, when the anti-nausea drug thalidomide slipped past all the safeguards to cause untold damage, both in pain and suffering for the children born without limbs and in anguish and guilt for the women who took this approved medication during their pregnancies. And they are also criticized when they do what they are mandated to do—oversee and regulate all aspects of drug testing, from the first issue of an Investigational New Drug (IND) permit to phase 3 clinical trials and full release of the drug into the market. Critics say they are overzealous, biased, vindictive, and in bed with big business. A former special assistant to the FDA's commissioner wrote to the *Washington Times* in 1995 that "There is a rewards-and-punishment system at FDA and . . . retaliation is very much a way of life" (Elias 1997, p. 27).

Supporters say such controls as clinical trials protect the very foundations of medical science. The danger of "unproven" therapies—that is, unproven on the ladder of scientific testing, first in the laboratory, then in several stages of clinical trials—is that they attract people away from conventional approaches that have been through the process. But for cancer patients who have "failed" such treatment, that "proven" track record is a house of cards that has collapsed under the real test, the only proof for them—their own individual experience.

It is an old debate, as old as government itself, inextricably linked with medical practices through the ages. Since the marriage of science and medicine through clinical trials, the fine line between government tyranny and genuine protection of citizens has become, in some minds, as bright and sharp and convincing as a scalpel, for others, a distinction lost in a thicket of politics, religion, and commerce. It is a debate operating on two levels: the right to provide treatment unsanctioned by regulatory agencies, and the right to seek it. The story of the temporary closure of the IAT Clinic in 1985 contains all the issues of this debate. However murky the facts and the motivations of the players, one thing is absolutely clear: the action of a bureaucracy killed people as surely as a quack wielding a surgical knife.

For the Tufaros the story started in April 1982. Theresa Tufaro's mother had just been diagnosed with malignant melanoma. The doctors had painted a "horrible, horrible picture . . . malignant melanoma is the most treacherous of cancers, the most painful way of dying and that was [my mother's] biggest fear. . . . The surgeon said, 'We have nothing to offer, there is no chemo, there is no radiation. She will not see the holidays.' At first we thought he meant Christmas—it turned out he meant the summer holidays. My father sat us down, we were four daughters, he said, 'Everywhere in the world, we must research, find alternatives, call every possible organization.' I had heard of something in the Bahamas, but I couldn't remember anything else. My prayers were every night, 'Just lead us in the right direction and we'll do what we have to do but we need You to lead us because we don't have time, we don't have time.'

"I called the IAT Clinic, I called all night long and finally someone answered. . . . I said, 'I need to speak to Dr. Burton,' but I was told, 'Dr Burton can't speak to you, there are too many patients and people for him to speak to everyone. . . .' Dr. Burton called me back the next day and he spoke to me for two hours."

Within two days of Theresa's conversation with Dr. Burton, her mother was on a flight to Freeport. "We took her without permission from the hospital. . . . she had her stitches still, but with the doctors saying she had only three to four months to live, you don't hang around. . . . When Burton met her, he said, 'Look at you, I see the fear all over your face, you're going to be fine, trust me.'"

She did, and she was, for four years.

Well before Burton moved his clinic to Freeport, about the time he came squarely into the cross-hairs of the Big Guns of the medical establishment, he began to find it harder and harder to get his research published. By 1971, he gave up trying: "I'm not in it for public money so I won't publish." Critics said he did not want to share his findings, that he was secretive and paranoid. This accusation was made often enough that a cartoon hangs in the clinic to this day: "Even paranoids have enemies."

Burton quoted the advice of Dr. Sidney Farber, a prominent chemotherapist of the time, on his decision not to try and publish anything anymore: "Look, you're ten to twenty years ahead of your time. You've got three options. First, you can keep repeating the same work over and over. Or second, you can keep rewriting and resubmitting your papers. Or third, you can keep chopping wood—just keep working and forget what's going on around you" (Moss 1996, p. 244; Wright 1985, p. 48; Anderson 1974, p. 46).

Burton chose option three.

The wood chopping ended suddenly one July day in 1985, when Burton received a letter from the Bahamian health authorities instructing him to close the clinic and stop treating patients immediately. The charge: the IAT serum was contaminated with the AIDS virus.

This was the year AIDS became a media epidemic in North America. The very word evoked fear and misunderstanding wherever it was heard, not least among the IAT patients. Now they believed that not only were they fighting cancer, they had AIDS to deal with as well. This sad chapter of the IAT saga reads like overheated fiction. Accusations of intrigue, bribery, and lying zing throughout the tale and have their echoes still in some quarters. Although the clinic was completely exonerated, and even its most voluble critics admitted that the blood product was not contaminated, the impact of the charge is still felt today.

Briefly the story is this: an IAT patient, Mary Anna Good of Tacoma, Washington, saw a letter by Dr. Curt of the NCI published in the *New England Journal of Medicine* claiming that the serum of four IAT patients had tested positive for hepatitis B. Period. The letter offered no other details, such as that this was not unusual, since the entire U.S. blood supply at the time was contaminated with hepatitis B. The Centers for Disease Control that same year noted that "tests of immune globulin lots prepared since 1977 indicate that both types of antibody [hepatitis A and hepatitis B] have been uniformly present" (CDC 1985). The letter worried Ms. Good, prompting her to take vials of IAT serum to be tested at the Tacoma–Pierce County Blood Bank. The first results indicated that all the samples tested positive for hepatitis antibodies and eight of the eighteen samples tested positive for HIV antibodies. Lab reports obtained under the Freedom of Information Act by a Washington attorney read, "None of these are strong positives, only C-1 has any real strength and it's only .3 above the cutoff" (Moss 1996, p. 262).

The immunoassay method used to test for HIV antibodies, known as ELISA (enzyme-linked immunosorbent assay), had been licenced for use only two months before; until then no testing kit had been commercially available. And one of the problems with the new method was that it often gave false positive results. Approximately 75 percent of U.S. tests results showing an initial positive reading by one kit turned out to be negative (Null and Steinman 1986).

The serum was then sent to the Centers for Disease Control for confirmation testing by both the immunoassay and the more accurate test, the Western Blot method, which indicated that all the samples tested negative. But this information was not released. "The CDC . . . and Dr. Curt at the NCI knew that the more specific test to confirm [the] findings, the Western Blot, was negative. This was in their own documents. . . . We did not create these documents. I think that speaks for itself" (United States 1986; testimony of Patrick McGrady, Sr., vice-president of the American Ageing Association, scientific adviser to the NW Oncology Foundation, and member of the Medical Advisory Board of the NW chapter of the American Medical Writers Association, at Guy Molinari hearing). Nor did it deter the CDC and PAHO (Pan American Health Organization) from sending a joint team to meet Bahamian officials and inspect the IAT Clinic in early July 1985. According to Burton, the team spent less than ten minutes on site. Two weeks later, his clinic was closed down.

It was a bad time for IAT patients. Unable to get their serum, they were frightened, some of them to death. The reported number of IAT patients who died during the eight months the clinic was closed range from thirty to sixty. On the July day when a handwritten note was pinned to the locked doors of the clinic announcing its closure, Frank Wiewel and his wife, Joanne, were in Freeport with her father, who was being treated for colon cancer. They went into high gear and, with several other patients and their families, gathered information and talked, or tried to talk, to all the officials involved in the shutdown. They eventually took their case to Washington.

Theresa Tufaro was there with her mother and father. "We really didn't understand what was going on. We only knew that my mother couldn't get her serum and we needed to have the clinic open. My mother and father helped organize the trip to Washington—my father hired buses for patients, and our motto became 'IAT, the Intelligent Alternative Therapy.'"

The IAT patients were warmly received on Capitol Hill. Congressman Guy V. Molinari of Staten Island, New York, was sufficiently interested to visit the Bahamas both to try and speak with Bahamian officials about the closure (they wouldn't discuss it) and to meet Burton. The result was a congressional public hearing which was described by one writer as "an epochal event in the struggle for freedom of choice in cancer [treatment]" (Moss 1996, p. 267). Held in New York in January 1986, the hearing presents a picture of the seamier side and long reach of medical politics.

Congressman Molinari opened with the following words:

There is a story collected in those present which desperately needs to be told. It involves Dr. Lawrence Burton, a researcher who developed an experimental cancer treatment called Immuno-Augmentative Therapy (IAT), whose clinic in Freeport, Grand Bahama, was forcibly closed last July by the Bahamian Government for reasons that remain unclear.

It also involves the many hundreds of cancer patients who were receiving treatment at that clinic and who now believe that their last hope for fighting their disease has been unfairly yanked away from them.

In my investigation I have found inconsistencies, and in some cases actual untruths, on the part of various agencies which I contacted, especially on the part of Dr. Gregory Curt of the NCI. (United States 1986).

While the IAT patients were in Washington, Theresa said they were told by some of the news media, "This is a very big cover-up, a very big political cover-up." As she describes the events twelve years after, her voice hardens with anger. "After three and a half years of being perfectly healthy while on [IAT] treatment, after two months without it, in September [my mother] developed on her chest a little black mark . . . It was the melanoma back. Then in January she was washing her face and noticed what she thought was mascara on the inside of her eyelid. She tried to wash it away and it wouldn't come off. Of course, it was melanoma. . . . My mother just started going downhill so fast."

The IAT Clinic was allowed to reopen two months after the hearings, two weeks after Theresa's mother died.

The cancer patients at the IAT Clinic had left their own country to exercise their freedom of choice in cancer treatment. They were not breaking the rules. Dr. Burton had left his own country to exercise his freedom of choice in providing a therapy he and many others believed in, a treatment that had no deleterious side effects, a treatment for which there was at least anecdotal evidence that it helps to control cancer. He was not breaking the rules. Yet the long arm of the U.S. regulatory agencies had apparently reached beyond their jurisdiction, persuading others to join in curtailing that freedom of choice. Some would defend their actions, saying that they were acting for the public good; others would say that there is evidence of a vendetta, the seeds of which were planted in the early skirmishes between Burton and the Acronyms.

Whatever other certainties surface out of the murk of this episode, there is the incontrovertible fact of the deaths of many people who believed that their lives depended on their access to the IAT serum. Whether science eventually "proves" that their lives depended on the treatment itself or only on the hope it provided is not the issue here. Rather, it is one that all cancer patients face—the issue of their right to choose a particular therapy, a particular route to hope.

Down the history of medicine, the most dramatic leaps forward, rather than sideways or in circles, are made by the philosophers, the scientists, the doctors who looked beyond the status quo. Dr. Burton looked beyond the status quo and was branded a maverick in an environment that shows little tolerance for individuals who don't toe the line. He marched to his own drummer and trampled all over that line. The price for his intransigence was exile and the label of quack.

Brewer's *Dictionary of Phrase and Fable* defines a quack as a "puffer of salves; an itinerant drug vendor at fairs who 'quacked' forth the praises of his wares to the credulous rustics." Another derivation suggests that the term may come from the Dutch "quacksalver" meaning quicksilver doctor, referring to mercury, which was widely used for centuries as an ointment applied to syphilis patients' ulcerations and sores, with drastic side effects and little impact on the disease. Whatever the derivation, "quack" is a favorite epithet used to blacken the reputations of doctors or scientists who work outside the medical mainstream.

Certainly, there are "quicksilver doctors" out there, but they are not unique to the territory beyond the boundaries of the medical establishment. Quacks and frauds turn up everywhere; but when they are flushed out of the thickets of traditional medicine they are usually assumed to be innocent until proven guilty. Cases pop up regularly of "doctors" who have been plying their trade in prestigious hospitals for years. When the rumors start, these individuals are usually defended vigorously by their professional organizations until the record of botched surgeries, drug overdoses, evidence of incompetence and unprofessional conduct, complaints from patients, and finally just too many deaths on their watch mount too high to be discounted.

But practitioners and proponents of alternative cancer therapies are considered guilty of quackery by association; their very profession makes them suspect. They are guilty until proven innocent, often decades, sometimes centuries, after their time.

The stories of other mavericks who stand outside the doors of the establishment are remarkably similar to Dr. Burton's— scientists and doctors who have attracted the wrath of the medical establishment and its regulatory agencies, exiled in the name of protection of cancer patients. Like Burton, Stanislaw Burzynski, a doctor and cancer researcher in Texas, also ran afoul of the FDA. He tried to play by its rules but wanted to develop and bring to market his cancer drug on his own without involving anyone else. He believed it was safe and effective without side effects and that patients should not have to wait years for it to go through the FDA process before having access to it. "This is the sort of action the FDA considers an end run around its usually useful anti-snake oil regulations" (Elias 1997, p. 27). The price for Dr. Burzynski's independence was fourteen years of legal fights and the label of quack.

Educated in Poland, where he was one of the two youngest people in that country with both M.D. and Ph.D. degrees, Dr. Burzynski came to the United States in 1970 to continue his research on blood peptides at the Baylor College of Medicine in Houston, Texas.

A few years later he set up his own small clinic and laboratory, working on "antineoplastons," a term he coined to describe the peptides he had isolated in the blood and urine which apparently had anticancer properties. The word "neoplasm" is the Greek term for a cancer tumor, literally "new growth." "Antineoplaston" simply means "anticancer."

Dr. Burzynski's history with the FDA began innocuously enough. In 1977 he asked the agency if it objected to his making antineoplastons and using them in the state of Texas. Absolutely not, the agency said. Then he checked with the Texas attorney general's office, which also gave him the green light.

In 1978, an FDA inspector checked his lab and asked for minor modifications. Burzynski complied and did not hear from the FDA for another four years. He treated about thirty new patients a year during this time.

By 1982, officialdom was closing in. Favorable media reports had brought Burzynski to the attention of Canadian health regulators, including the Ontario Medical Association, which sent experts to review the treatment. The outcome was remarkably similar to that of the medical teams sent to assess Burton's work. Thumbs down. They claimed that they could see no evidence of efficacy in the use of antineoplastons against cancer, and the Ontario Hospital Insurance Program (OHIP) stopped paying claims made by Canadian patients going to Burzynski.

The Canadian authorities sent samples of antineoplastons to the American NCI for testing, and shortly afterward the FDA was on his doorstep again, this time for several weeks.

In Easter week, 1983, the FDA filed its lawsuit against him, and the war was on. It took twelve years to get him to trial: the first FDA injunction was quashed by a federal judge, and by 1988 two federal grand juries had refused to indict him. In 1995, the FDA finally got charges to stick, but they were not for malpractice or quackery; they were for contempt of court, insurance fraud, and interstate commerce of an unapproved drug. But by then his drug *was* approved, at least for human tests. By the time his case went to trial in early January 1997, Burzynski had been granted sixty-nine IND permits by the same agency that was trying to nail him for quackery.

This inconsistency did not prevent proceedings. In his opening remarks, the judge made it clear that it was Burzynski and not his drug that was on trial: "Whether or not any patient or former patient believes Dr. Burzynski's drug is effective is not going to be an issue. We are not going to hear evidence of whether any drug or treatment offered by [Burzynski] is effective or not" (Elias 1997, p. 29).

This might be good law, but it is astonishing logic. For those who are fighting cancer, it was the cock-eyed "off-with-his-head" justice of Alice's Queen. Whether the drug worked was the *only* issue. Otherwise, why was this man on trial at all? Either he was a quack, making false claims for a drug that was useless, bilking his patients, selling false hope—and across state lines, at that. Or he wasn't. And if he wasn't, or if that wasn't the charge, then there was no case. His first trial in 1997 ended with a hung jury. The second one, two months later, didn't. It took the jury less than three hours to acquit him.

It is difficult to characterize this saga as anything more than a vendetta on the part of the government, "a Big Brother issue," as a jury member later described it. However, the prosecuting lawyer had a different take: "It concerns me as a government employee to see a trend toward government bashing, and this was part of it."

The FDA had been after Burzynski for fourteen years. Its lawyers had shown their hand in the very first hearing in 1985: "If this court declines to grant the injunctive relief sought by the government, thus permitting continued manufacturing and distribution of antineoplastons by [Burzynski] in violation of the Food, Drug and Cosmetic Act, the government then would be obliged to pursue other, less efficient remedies" (Elias 1997, p. 160). The court declined, the government resorted to "less efficient remedies," and lost. It would seem odd to characterize these events as "government bashing."

But the fourteen-year fight took its toll. Much of the medical establishment still sees Burzynski as a quack. He made the same mistake as Burton did: he stands firm in his beliefs about cancer and the way it works, beliefs that contradict those of "the scientific priesthood," as his one-time research partner, Dr. Carlton Hazlewood at the Baylor College of Medicine, called them.

The career of Dr. Gaston Naessens, a French scientist now living in Canada, is pockmarked by the salvos of authorities in three countries. His crime? "Dabbling in healing," as one observer described it. The price he paid for his unorthodox views was fines, arrests, exile, and a trial for contributing to the death of a patient. And the label of quack. His trial, unlike Burzynski's, was very much grounded on the question of the efficacy of his anticancer product, 714-X. If it worked, he was not a quack. If it didn't, he was.

In the 1940s, in France, Dr. Naessens developed a microscope with extraordinarily powerful magnification and resolution, a version of what is now known as dark-field microscopy. Naessens's subsequent studies of human blood with this microscope, which "reveal[ed] with spectacular clarity the motion and multiplicity of . . . organisms in the blood" (Sloan-Kettering scientist quoted in Roberts 1992, p. 96), led him to develop 714-X, a non-toxic product designed to prevent the replication of cancer cells.

He was chased out of Europe when complaints from some pharmacists and physicians that this "uncredentialled young biologist was dabbling in healing" (ibid., p. 57) led to fines and closure of his lab. He came to Canada and in 1971, with private backing, opened a lab in Montreal; he subsequently moved to the Eastern Townships where his backer thought he would attract less attention from the orthodox medical community. It was not to be. "His run-ins with the medical authorities in

France had forever branded him a quack; his name was on the Quebec Medical Corporation's blacklist" (ibid.).

Although medical scientists were interested in pursuing Naessens's work, the medical bureaucracy was not. At one point in the mid-1970s a team from the Memorial Sloan-Kettering Cancer Center came to his lab and was enormously impressed, especially with his microscope, the implications of which "are staggering. . . . It is imperative that what its inventor, a dedicated biological scientist, is doing and can do, be totally reviewed. I am convinced that he is an authentic genius and that his achievements cut across and illumine some of the most pertinent areas of medical science" (ibid., p. 96). The team urged Sloan-Kettering to bring Naessens to work at the Center, but when it was pointed out that he was on the American Cancer Society's "blacklist," the recommendations of the team of expert scientists were overruled by the bureaucrats. Naessens was back to "chopping wood" in the backwaters of Quebec, where a growing number of patients found him. In 1984, so did the Quebec police. His lab was raided and his files and vials were seized. In 1989 he was tried for illegal practice of medicine and contributing to the death of a patient.

"Witness after witness took the stand to describe the horrors of their battles with cancer and the apparent cures they'd finally achieved after using Naessens' treatment" (ibid., p. 52). And Naessens's integrity shone through the testimonies: he had never promised a cure, never encouraged anyone to discontinue conventional treatment, and never asked for payment. He was acquitted on all charges. The head of the Quebec Medical Corporation, Dr. Augustin Roy, was enraged. An article in *Saturday Night* magazine quotes him as saying that the prosecutor should have "savagely cross-examined everyone of the patients who had testified on Naessens' behalf," that they "simply don't know the difference between *feeling* healthy and *being* healthy. . . . All of them should stand at attention or, more properly, get down on their knees to thank orthodox medicine for having kept them alive" (ibid., p. 54).

Quacks are most often exposed through an accumulation of complaints from patients. In the cases of Burton, of Burzynski, and of Naessens, it is the opposite. The charges of quackery and fraud were brought against these three men by their "peers." Their patients and the people taking their therapies are their most vigorous defenders, traveling to the seat of political power to plead their case, and picketing courtrooms and news agencies in their defense. It is remarkable how similar their stories are. Three highly educated, experienced researchers start out in the mainstream and after years of work proffer theories and therapies that run counter to the accepted direction of cancer treatment. In the end all three are vilified.

These three men, and there are many others, have suffered greatly because they have been labeled "quacks." Yet none of them fits the description given by the bureaucrats of the establishment: they do not claim to have the ultimate cure for cancer; they do not lure patients away from conventional treatments in an either/or tussle; they do not profess to have a "secret ingredient" tantamount to the elixir of life; and they do not charge exorbitant fees.

It seems, rather, that the crimes of these alternative practitioners are of another nature. They have each arrived, through scientific research, at theories that do not fit within the parameters of current treatment approaches. They are medical heretics, perhaps, but hardly "puffers of salves" or "quicksilver doctors."

In a United States hospital, a twenty-year-old woman is suffering from aplastic anaemia. Because of her religious beliefs—the young woman is a Jehovah's Witness—she refuses blood transfusions, the only procedure that would save her life. She is unshakeable in her conviction despite her doctors' pleas. "I talked blood transfusions every day. I've never been so frustrated in my life. I teach in the medical ethics program here. Our position is always that the patient's beliefs must be honored. But it was so difficult" (Roueché 1996, p. 72). The young woman died.

She was allowed the right *not* to choose a procedure that the doctors knew would have saved her life. The patients taking the therapies of Burton, Burzynski, and Naessens, and the patients at the Tijuana clinics, those on cancer vaccines or megavitamin therapy, are asking for the right to choose a medical intervention they believe will help them live. They would ask: "Where is the difference? She had the freedom of choice to risk death. We ask only for the freedom of choice to risk living."

It would seem that you are free to make medical choices as long as you stay within the corridors of mainstream medicine; you can go through any of the doors opening off those corridors except the one that leads out of the building.

Sherwin Nuland, a surgeon and author of *Doctors: The Biography of Medicine*, has a theory about medical progress: timing is all. "When the cultural milieu is just right . . . when enough restless minds have begun to chafe under the status quo, some one spunky spirit comes forward to deliver the enlightening goods" (1995, p. 239). He is referring to specific giants of medicine, "the . . . 'great docs' history which celebrate[s] the triumphal progress of medicine from ignorance through error to science" (Porter 1997a, p. 6). But medical progress doesn't soar forward in a single trajectory toward the ultimate perfect answers. It moves more like a wavery line of inchworms hauling their earnest little bodies two creeps forward, one creep back, in an erratic process of advances and retreats, mistakes, and breakthroughs. Some blunder down the many "blind alleys of medical research" (Nuland 1995, p. 240). Others blaze more promising trails, but even these will not lead to success unless society is ready for them.

In the last few years, interest in alternative therapies has skyrocketed. An Angus Reid poll published in the fall of 1997 says that almost 50 percent of adult Canadians now use some form of unconventional therapy, up from 10 percent only three years earlier. In the United States, a study of trends in alternative medicine between 1990 and 1997 found that use of at least one alternative therapy had increased from 33.8 percent to 42.1 percent (Fugh-Berman 1999a). Ranging from aromatherapy to Zen, acupuncture to fly fishing, energy balancing to herbal medicine, these therapies are being used to treat ailments from the common cold to cancer. Perhaps our society is preparing a more accommodating milieu for some of those inchworms of promise and progress.

Although the alternative and conventional cancer practitioners are not noticeably friendlier with each other, the rising interest in alternative cancer therapies and the fierce demands by patients for the right to use them have caused some thawing in the regulatory world.

In Canada, a Task Force on Alternative Therapies was set up under the aegis of the Canadian Breast Cancer Research Initiative, a federal project to look at essiac, hydrazine sulfate, green tea, Iscador, 714-X, and megadoses of vitamins A, C, and E. The results of these studies were published, not in the alternative popular press, but in the pages of the august *Canadian Medical Association Journal* (Kaegi 1998). They are refreshing in their carefully worded lack of condemnation.

Health Canada's Special Access Program within the Therapeutic Products Program (TPP), is responsible for authorizing the sale of pharmaceutical, biological, and radiopharmaceutical products that are not approved in Canada. Ian Mackay, head of the Special Access Program, says "they work in partnership with physicians and drug manufacturers to provide access to products not marketed in Canada for physicians treating patients with life-threatening conditions when conventional therapies have failed, are unsuitable or unavailable." The program does have discretionary powers, but it appears to see its role as a facilitator rather than a gatekeeper. "Generally speaking, what we are looking for is a clear rationale from a physician which states that the drug in question is the patient's only option," Mackay says. Health Canada then contacts the manufacturer to ensure that information about the drug is "well-described" and that any safety concerns about it are raised. "This review does not represent an opinion, statement or effort to determine that the drug is safe, efficacious or of high quality." In other words, Buyer Beware.

Promising developments elsewhere in Canada include the Centre for Integrated Healing which opened in Vancouver in April 1999 under the direction of Dr. Roger Rogers and Dr. Hal Gunn. The Centre provides both information on and access to alternative cancer therapies, at the same time enjoying a good supportive relationship with the British Columbia government and the provincial cancer agency: it is partially funded by the British Columbia Medical Services Plan with supervision by the British Columbia Cancer Agency. Dr. Simon Surcliffe, the agency's Vancouver region vice-president, says, "The public clearly wants alternative medicine options, and we are keen to learn what constitutes a quality complementary experience. We are satisfied that funding the centre is a good way to start learning and evaluating the efficiency of this approach to treating cancer" (Maser 1999, p. 43).

The Centre believes that conventional medical treatment can play a valuable role in the recovery from cancer but that it is just one spoke in the wheel of an integrated holistic approach to healing. "The bio-medical model perceives 'illness' as separate from 'self' and thus . . . can be treated with outside agents (e.g., surgery, radiation, chemotherapy). There is rapidly growing evidence from the field of psychoneuroimmunologists that this view of illness is very limited, and that illness and our immune system are not separate from 'self' . . . that our mind and our body are inseparable and that healing and the healthy functioning of our immune system involve much more than simple medical treatments" (Centre for Integrated Healing 1999, p. 4).

In the United States, the Office for the Study of Unconventional Medical Practices, renamed the Office of Alternative Medicine (OAM), was set up within the National Institutes of Health in 1992. The creation of such an office within an organization described by the *Sunday Times* as the "stern protector of the most rigorous brand of science" looked like progress, but within a year it was adrift on a sea of internal fighting. One step forward, two steps back. Berkley Bedell, a retired Democratic congressman from Iowa, was one of the movers behind the formation of the OAM. "When alternative treatments appeared to cure my Lyme disease and prostate cancer, which had caused me to retire after twelve years in the United States Congress, I decided that my main mission in life would be that such treatments are properly investigated."

Fed up with the delays and posturing within the OAM, particularly in its field investigations, Bedell launched his own National Foundation for Alternative Medicine (NFAM) in 1998. The goal of this non-profit organization is to investigate and report on "what clinical research evidence suggests to be the most promising alternative treatments being administered around the world for various health problems" and to collect and disseminate "information on the experiences of those who use such treatments" (NFAM brochure).

The National Cancer Institute appears to be taking a more open position on alternative approaches. At a hearing before the House Committee on Government Reform in June 1999, Edward L. Trimble, head of Surgery Section, Division of Cancer Treatment and Diagnosis at the NCI, spoke of the role of alternative medicine in the detection and treatment of women's cancers. Following the *de rigueur* good-news pronouncements—"Our Nation is experiencing real progress against cancer. . . ."—he announced that "we have taken steps to significantly alter our approaches to complementary and alternative medicine" (Trimble 1999, p. 1).

These altered approaches include cosponsoring a phase 3 trial with the National Center for Complementary and Alternative Medicine (NCCAM) on shark cartilage, and "moving ahead" with an evaluation of nutritional therapies, the therapeutic value of vitamins and minerals, and possibly even a study of green tea as a cancer prevention strategy.

In July 1999, the long-awaited Cancer Advisory Panel on Complementary and Alternative Medicine (CAPCAM) was formally launched by the National Institutes of Health, in collaboration with the NCI. Its members will advise on the merits of clinical trials involving alternative cancer therapies, determine research opportunities, and develop methods of communicating the results.

The panel will "review and evaluate summaries of evidence for CAM [Complementary and Alternative Medicine] cancer claims submitted by practitioners" (ibid.). Private-sector competition may have helped get this panel up and running: its mandate sounds remarkably like that of Bedell's organization.

The IAT Clinic; along with other legitimate alternative therapy clinics and practitioners, welcomes such developments. But after being promised since 1991 that its therapy would be fairly assessed, the clinic staff response is measured. The best-case records still wait on a desk in the record room. Perhaps it will happen this year.

The patients at IAT aren't holding their breath either. They don't need official words to tell them about the therapy they see as having protected them so far. Once you are in the world of cancer, the debates, assessments, conferences, committee hearings, legislation, lobbying, and lallygagging are distant thunder in the middle of the night when it is just you, alone, with your disease.

10

Cancer Treatment's Bottom Line: Cash or Cure?

In the debate about cancer treatments, you will certainly hear about cancer as Big Business. The current lingo underlines the view that cancer is not a disease but a commodity; sick people are not patients but "health consumers." People who need treatment, who need their health insurance to cover those treatments, who are persuaded into clinical trials, are not patients but "clients." If cancer were on the stock market, it would be a good buy.

You hear the argument that freedom of medical choice is restricted not to protect citizens, but to protect the almighty dollar. It goes like this: Cancer is just another industry, with the market determining the direction of treatment and research. Since the production of cancer treatment drugs—chemotherapies—is such a lucrative enterprise, their producers block other therapies that are cheaper to produce, unpatentable and which could threaten the profits or market share of what are sometimes called "ethical" pharmaceuticals (AstraZeneca web site).

The economic argument is certainly compelling. The cancer industry, indeed the entire health industry, is a tangle of vested interests including the pharmaceutical companies, the health insurance agencies, the regulatory agencies, governments, lobbyists, and professional medical associations. It would be more surprising if these organizations did *not* fight to protect their market, given that, for example, the chemotherapy industry alone generates about $12 to $14 billion a year in the United States alone. But to what length and whose cost?

Stephanie Cosgrave was diagnosed with breast cancer two years ago. The tumor was small, contained, and carved out successfully. No need for any other treatment, her doctors said. Two years later the cancer was back. Even though the tumor exhibited the same tidy attributes, Stephanie didn't mess around. She had a double mastectomy with reconstruction and went into high-gear research mode, including attendance at the Second World Conference on Breast Cancer, held in Ottawa in July 1999. She was looking for some firm information on follow-up treatment of any kind—alternative, conventional, she didn't care. Tamoxifen was certainly one of her options, but the debate about the drug had her spinning. She had heard the arguments that it was absolutely the best breast cancer treatment available, a magic bullet, a wonder drug. You mean for treatment or for prevention? she asked. For both, was the reply.

Then she started hearing the other side of the debate. Dr. Samuel Epstein, professor of occupational and environmental medicine at the School of Public Health, University of Illinois Medical Center, Chicago, was one of the plenary speakers at the conference. A vociferous critic of the cancer establishment, and a lightning rod for its wrath, he believes that chemoprevention of breast cancer with tamoxifen is "an exercise in disease substitution rather than disease prevention." The pharmaceutical company Zeneca Inc. is the sole producer of the drug, under the registered trade name Nolvadex, and provided its product free of charge for the prevention trials. The drug's approval by the Food and Drug Administration (FDA) as a preventative therapy opened up a huge new market for Zeneca. Surely the FDA's approval is assurance that tamoxifen is safe and a good bet for women at risk for developing breast cancer or for preventing a recurrence? Not necessarily. The FDA hedged its bets, allowing Zeneca to market it as a drug that would "reduce the risk" of breast cancer, not that would "prevent breast cancer." The medical oncologist at Zeneca dismissed this as so much semantic nonsense, saying cheerfully on a CBC-TV interview that doctors, when they prescribed the drug, could still tell women it prevented breast cancer.

For Stephanie, this is not semantic nonsense, it is a semantic nightmare—especially now that the waters are muddied with the suspicion that it is all just big business anyway. Then she heard about raloxifene, a second generation of a group of drugs known as "selective estrogen receptor modulators," or SERMs, of which tamoxifen is first generation. This drug, marketed as Evista and manufactured by Eli Lilly, appears not to pose risks of uterine cancer, as does tamoxifen, and has already been approved for treatment of osteoporosis. Its arrival on the breast cancer treatment scene was heralded by the media as a breakthrough: yet another one. Not everyone agrees.

Dr. Epstein writes that Lilly's claims about the drug's efficacy in breast cancer prevention are based on two small studies involving fewer than fifty women (1998, p. 489). Such a slim foundation, plus the anecdotal evidence arising from its osteoporosis studies, was enough evidence for Lilly to launch a marketing campaign including a fact sheet for doctors that reads: "Evista prevents osteoporosis, lowers 'bad' cholesterol," and "reduces the incidence of breast cancer." Based on the same evidence, the American National Cancer Institute has announced a huge "head to head" prevention trial (the Star trial) comparing tamoxifen and raloxifene, involving 22,000 well women.

This evidence was not enough to convince its competitor, Zeneca, which promptly filed a suit against Eli Lilly for false advertising. And won. A New York District Court issued a preliminary injunction in July 1999, preventing Eli Lilly from claiming that its drug reduces the risk of breast cancer. So what does this do to the Star trial? Apparently nothing. The recruitment of women to enter the trial continues. So now Stephanie hears about this market-share / public-relations war raging between the rival manufacturers of the two drugs, which raises a huge question in Stephanie's mind. Are they in it for me, and all the other women in this world with breast cancer, or are they in it for the money, pure and simple?

But then Stephanie hears even more disturbing claims and wonders if they are just the rants and rails of malcontents and paranoids, or truthful reports from mavericks and whistle-blowers whose lonely voices manage to pierce the establishment choir. Their message is one of conspiracy, the Big Business scenario taken a dark step further, and it goes like this: An entire industry rests on cancer not being beaten. If a cure were found, particularly a non-pharmaceutical cure, the walls would come tumbling down, thousands of people would be out of work. Big Money interests would collapse.

After World War II, the military industrial interests had to look for another base or implode: the military–medical marriage was born, with much of the technology and chemical research re-targeted on cancer as the new enemy. If the war on cancer were won, this entangled world of vested interests would unravel, causing a paradigm shift of similar seismic proportions.

Paul Schubert thought about this a lot while he was trying to decide what direction to go when faced with the bleak track record of chemotherapy with colon cancer: "There is an old theory that if you want to find out why things are as they are follow the money to the source. You can get into a real heavy discussion about how big the business of cancer is. Follow that back to the drug companies. The cost of this treatment [IAT] compared to chemotherapy is minuscule. They were talking of having me on chemo for six months, something like that, every couple of weeks for six months. That would be $100,000. For something that they know isn't going to work. But it really is big business. Millions of dollars a year are generated. Think about all of the jobs. If cancer didn't exist would we need as many medical professionals as we have now? You wouldn't need the National Cancer Institute or the American Cancer Society. A lot of the drug companies wouldn't need to be producing the chemo so therefore who knows what it would do to their income. . . ."

Dr. Epstein says that he has been investigating the American Cancer Society for three decades, and "I have very detailed documentation on [its] indifference, if not hostility, to cancer prevention" (plenary speech, Second World Conference on Breast Cancer, 1999). He criticizes such organizations for refusing to put the blame for the rising incidence of cancer where he feels it squarely belongs—with the chemical companies that put carcinogens in everything we ingest—the food we eat, the air we breathe, the water we drink. Instead of prevention, they support highly lucrative treatment modalities such as chemotherapies, and the mammography industry with its enormous market for machinery, film, and "clients" made captive by government programs urging women to "prevent" breast cancer by having a mammogram every year.

This interpretation feeds into another really depressing take on the whole cancer world. The companies that are busily developing drugs to treat cancer are the very ones that may be causing the disease in the first place. Zeneca, a huge pharmaceutical company and offshoot of Imperial Chemicals Industries, one of the world's largest pesticides manufacturers, is the sole manufacturer of tamoxifen. Zeneca is huge indeed: it is part of AstraZeneca PLC, one of the top five pharmaceutical companies in the world based on sales, a US$15.8 billion international bioscience business involved in the whole gamut: the research, development, manufacture, and marketing of pharmaceuticals and agricultural products. In the United States it also supplies health care services through Salik Health Care. When a company has fingers in so many pies, consumers can only wonder if the left hand knows what the right is doing.

Activists point out that Du Pont and General Electric, which compete for the dubious distinction of having the highest number of hazardous waste sites in the United States, are the big players in the mammography business. GE makes the machines; Du Pont makes much of the film for those machines (Paulsen 1994). Both aggressively market mammography to younger women, despite the continuing controversy over the health hazards of regular exposure to low-level radiation. Tails you lose, heads you lose again. Either way, you are one of the cogs that keep the system ratcheting along.

In the conspiracy theory, the players are the same as in the economic scenario, but with the added murk of their hidden connections: pharmaceutical companies, the powerful research and treatment centers such as Sloan-Kettering with their alleged links with industry, insurance companies, and the nuclear power industry, all of which are in bed with government, the regulatory agencies, and the big cancer organizations such as the American and Canadian cancer societies. The fine hands of the lobbyists knit and purl the interlinking skeins of power between government and industry. A recent example was the defeat of legislation in the U.S. Senate in 1999 that would have allowed doctors rather than health insurance companies to determine length of hospital stay for women following mastectomies or other surgeries for breast cancer.

Dr. Epstein calls it the politics of cancer, and urges everyone to check out the nacreous underbelly of science and treatment choices. He points out that the policies governing cancer research and treatment are guided by such powerful entities as the American Cancer Society (ACS), the National Cancer Institute (NCI), and the Food and Drug Administration (FDA), which he claims are in direct conflict of interest. He quotes former NCI director Samuel Broder as saying that the NCI has become "what amounts to a governmental pharmaceutical company." The NCI, he says, has—with enthusiastic support from the ACS—effectively blocked funds for research and clinical trials of promising non-toxic alternative cancer drugs for decades in favor of highly toxic and largely ineffective patented drugs developed by the big pharmaceutical companies.

This kind of talk drives the establishment crazy: Dr. Elizabeth Whelan, president of the American Council on Science and Health, calls him "way off the map. He is just so far out of the mainstream. It's absurd." (*Ottawa Citizen*, July 29, 1999). Well, yes, there's no denying he's out of step with much of the cancer treatment world, but for many who heard him speak at the conference, or who have read his book on the politics of cancer, that only adds to his credibility. His claims about blocked research and fair trials are bolstered by the sorry history of the attempts to have such alternative therapies as IAT, 714-X, and antineoplastons fairly assessed.

The IAT story is studded with hopeful plans for both clinical and field studies, all of which have come to naught. In 1986, Congressman Guy Molinari and twenty-three other members of Congress, as well as fourteen senators, formally requested the congressional Office of Technical Assessment (OTA) to conduct a formal study of IAT. When nothing had happened two years later, Burton and his team proposed to the OTA a three-stage evaluation process: a review of his clinic's records, a pre-trial of current IAT patients, and a full-scale randomized controlled trial in the United States (Moss 1996, p. xi). Even the first step of this proposal has not been acted upon. Despite the NCI's apparent progress in setting up an independent panel to look at alternative therapies, the records still sit in the file room at the IAT Clinic waiting for the promised review.

Burzynski began asking as early as 1981 for the NCI and the ACS to review his patient records, but neither would do it. (Elias 1997, p. 199). Finally, in 1991, NCI sent a team of scientists to conduct an on-site visit. They stayed one day, and agreed to take only seven best-response cases, although Burzynski urged them to take at least twenty brain tumor cases. Even so, their report was favorable—the team found "possible complete responses" in four of the seven cases and partial response (50 percent or more tumor reduction) in the other three. "So compelling were the results that Dr. Michael Friedman, then NCI associate director for the CTEP [Cancer Therapy Evaluation Program] and later acting FDA commissioner, wrote in an internal memo to the director of NCI's Division of Cancer Treatment that 'antineoplastons deserve a closer look. It turns out that the agents are well defined, pure chemical entities. . . . The human brain tumor responses are real. We will keep you informed'" (ibid., p. 200).

Nothing happened for two years. Finally, a three-site antineoplaston trial was set up for 1994–95, but it foundered on in-fighting and politics. Burzynski was excluded from receiving the results of the tests of his own drug, and the NCI changed the inclusion criteria and protocols, changes which Burzynski felt would threaten the accuracy of the trial. In the end, NCI canceled the trial.

Since 1990, Dr. Naessens's anticancer treatment, 714-X, has been available in Canada only through the Therapeutic Drug Program of Health Canada. Patients must have confirmed disease before a prescription is provided. According to the Centre d'Orthobiologie Somatidienne de l'Estrie Inc. (COSE), Naessens's organization, American citizens can obtain 714-X for either treatment of existing disease or as a preventive with a doctor's prescription (COSE 1990). These are hard to come by, however, and many patients told me they had been informed by their doctors that 714-X was illegal in the United States. Berkley Bedell's push to get alternative treatments fairly evaluated was partly based on his interest in 714-X, which he credits for his recovery from prostate cancer. Dr. Naessens would welcome a fair evaluation of his methods: "We . . . appreciate the efforts of Mr. Bedell and many others in trying to get alternative practices evaluated. We also understand the difficulties encountered by those trying to evaluate alternative treatments using orthodox methods (e.g., the double-blind study). . . . I want to reiterate that I myself am ready to cooperate with any investigations that I would consider honest and well-intentioned. But in my opinion, evaluation of alternative methods of intervention requires a different protocol of research than testing the effectiveness of the toxicity of a chemical compound" (Moss, 1994, p. 9).

The hounding of alternative therapies is not restricted to innuendo and delays in fair assessment of their efficacy. As the 1985 closing of the IAT Clinic demonstrates, the regulatory agencies can be more brutally direct and damaging than that. Ostensibly, the clinic was shut down because of an HIV/AIDS scare. Consider the context. In the mid-1980s, it was just being recognized that the entire blood supply, not only in the United States, but also in Canada and Europe, was compromised by both hepatitis strains and HIV. AIDS was surfacing throughout the western world. It was no longer a disease of developing countries but one on our own doorstep. Panic was mounting. And the fix was in. Federal agencies responsible for protecting public health were already practicing damage control. In February 1986, a letter in the *Journal of the American Medical Association* stated that people who received gamma globulin shots could test positive for HIV, even if they never became infected. *USA Today* (February 7, 1986) explained: "Gamma globulin is made from blood collected from thousands of donors . . . if just one donor has AIDS antibodies, the entire pool will test positive." But the FDA did not release this information right away because "we thought it would do more harm than good, since we saw no risk to the public health whatsoever [because] . . . in making gamma globulin, the AIDS virus itself is killed" (Moss 1996, p. 261).

Comforting but wrong. And in light of this reassurance to the public, why was the IAT Clinic targeted for something that was not, according to the FDA itself, a danger to health? Even as AIDS became more prevalent, and the full extent of the blood scandal surfaced, blood agencies, blood banks, clinics, and hospitals in the system were not shut down. As Dr. Clement explained: "I know of no other instance of the closing of a clinic, hospital or blood bank in this manner; in similar instances, the institutions are simply informed of the problem, they correct it, and go on" (United States 1986, Molinari hearing).

Testimony at this hearing revealed that of the fifty-six IAT patients who volunteered to be tested for HIV following the clinic closure, all tested negative; that there was not a single case of AIDS resulting from IAT treatment in five years; that the infectious-disease rate from IAT materials was lower than in any other U.S. or Bahamian facility; that no other health facility had been closed down as a result of similar tests; that the inspection by officials of the Pan-American Health

Organization and the Centers for Disease Control included no tests or evaluations that could substantiate a "serious health hazard"; that no official reasons were given for the clinic's closure; and that "threats were made" to Bahamian officials to encourage them to close the clinic. One Bahamian official implied that there had been discussions of the possible damage to the tourism industry of the islands if word got out of an AIDS epidemic sparked by a medical facility operating on their shores.

Rumors were flying, including at least one accusation of bribery in high places. An IAT patient who was at the clinic at the time said that Dr. Burton told her that the Bahamian authorities were paid to shut the clinic down. "Now Dr. Burton told me this story. . . . He said that the man who brought the money [from the States], the first $10,000, had brought a tape of the meeting [between the American and Bahamian officials] to Dr. B." This story never made it into the hearings summary.

Just as no official statement was made by the regulatory agencies officially explaining the closure, no official reason was given for permission for its reopening. But the damage was well and truly done. References to AIDS-contaminated serum still surface both in publications purporting to be unbiased data summaries and on the Internet web pages of the NCI and some Canadian cancer agencies. A random search turned up four web sites (including the Quackwatch page, the NCI page, the Ontario Breast Cancer Information Exchange Project, the British Columbia Cancer Agency, and the Atlantic Breast Cancer Information Exchange Project) still reporting claims that IAT serum is contaminated with bacteria, hepatitis, and HIV. Although claiming to be up to date (last update for the Canadian sites was given as 1997), nowhere do they report that these accusations were all proven to be false and the clinic exonerated—in 1986.

You are a cancer patient. Your chemotherapy treatments are not working. Or you are so sick on the treatment that you cannot face feeding more wretched down time into the hopper in the hopes that you get back a few days of living. You elect to investigate alternatives. You hear about the IAT Clinic from someone who has been there, who has been on the treatment, who is doing well. You read a couple of books on alternative therapies that describe IAT as a reasonable, well-researched approach to cancer control. Then you surf the Net to find that the treatment is suspect, it will probably give you AIDS, and Burton is making millions a year from gullible patients. Although he died in 1993, several web sites still have him living high off the hog. What do you *do* with this contradictory stuff? You spin. In the predawn hours you doubt, you despair, you struggle to make sense of the accusations and counter-accusations.

You must decide whether to believe that the regulatory authorities have spent years and millions of dollars to put Burton, Naessens, and Burzynski out of commission because they flog unproven cancer therapies to sick and vulnerable dupes, or because they crossed the wrong bureaucrat and thumbed their noses at the system that bureaucrat is charged with protecting. Burton's most ardent admirers admit that he could be arrogant, quick to anger, secretive, and paranoid. He did not help himself in official circles. And certainly Naessens appeared to have drawn the personal ire of Dr. Roy, who vowed not to give up after Naessens's acquittal. Within weeks, eighty-two more counts of practicing medicine without a license were brought against him.

You must decide whether these men are a threat to cancer *patients* or to the cancer *industry*, that it is not the failure of their therapies that is the problem, but their success. There is no question that the animosity continues. As recently as the

fall of 1999, mainstream research scientists agreed to be interviewed for this book only if they and their professional affil-
iations remained anonymous. They feared that any association
with IAT, even remote research and investigation of the com-
ponents of the serum, could bring down the wrath of such
bodies as Sloan-Kettering, and harm them professionally.
Theirs is not paranoia but a healthy instinct for survival.

For you, a cancer patient, these choices are not intellectual
exercises or an opportunity for debate but issues of life and
death. Your own. You must decide for yourself who is telling the
truth; if you opt for an alternative therapy, you must deal with
the fear that you might lose access to it at any time, because a
distant agency says so; you must wrestle with the planted nag
that maybe the therapy is useless because the authorities imply
or outright say so. You must deal with shaken faith, fading
hope, and energy dissipated not so much in your fight against
cancer as in your fight against the politics of cancer.

And the confusion and conflicts don't end there; they are
simply amplified by the media. One argument, an offshoot of
the Big Business theory, has it that: "Newspapers and broad-
casters very often depend on corporate press releases as unacknowledged sources for their 'news stories,' meaning that the
PR spin-doctors can clean up and slant adverse findings, and
promote fictitious 'good news' discoveries. The media abrogate
. . . [their] responsibility because competitive pressures have
left them without specialist staff who [can] bring knowledge
and cynicism to their reporting, and sometimes because they
need to mollify corporate advertisers. Often their . . . owners
will also have investments in the corporations or products . . ."
(Fist 1999).

The scuttlebutt here is that the old boys' network of media,
advertisers, and big business ensures that breakthroughs
within the establishment research community are reported

with frenzied excitement and distinct loss of perspective. Not always conscious propaganda, certainly, but effective nonetheless. For example, a report in the April 13, 1999, edition of *The National Post* caught the attention of Dr. Steven Narod, chair of breast cancer research at Women's College Hospital, Toronto. The headline announced a breakthrough in breast cancer treatment: a new drug, herceptin, increased survival by 22 percent. He was scathing. "Know what that means? It means a women who would be expected to live twelve months will now perhaps live thirteen months. And that's only 22 percent of women. The report says the disease is 'usually fatal until now.' Metastatic breast cancer still *is* fatal."

The mainstream media, on the other hand, generally treat with disdain—and alarming lack of primary research—positive developments in alternative cancer therapy treatment. There is an almost gleeful haste to write the debunking story, such as *Globe and Mail* columnist Margaret Wente's depiction of Tyrell Dueck's treatment at the American Biologics in Mexico: "In Tijuana, in a foreign land far from his friends and the place he loved, they hooked Tyrell up to an IV drip of apricot pits" (Wente 1999a). It is unlikely that this reporter would describe a Taxol treatment, a highly toxic but approved chemotherapy derived from the bark of the Pacific yew tree, as "being hooked up to an IV drip of tree bark." In a later column (July 31) she slammed the World Conference on Breast Cancer in Ottawa, although it is not clear whether she attended it. She cites, as an example of the ludicrous claims made at the conference, the belief that electromagnetic fields are linked with cancer. "As for power lines and electromagnetic fields, worry not. The links between this invisible force and various cancers have been studied for two decades. No one has been able to explain how these fields might cause cancer, and there's no convincing evidence that they're a health hazard." Yet even the mainstream media, her paper included, at the same time were publishing reports of research being done at the University of Toronto and the Hospital for Sick Children which was establishing that magnetic fields were indeed a health hazard. The research team has established a link between leukemia in children and exposure to magnetic and electrical fields. Later in that same column, Wente wrote, "The people who get hurt [by the "misinformation" emanating from critics of the establishment] are all the women who pick up a paper or listen to the radio or watch TV, and might half believe what they hear." Well, exactly.

Conspiracy, economics, vested interests, or biased media—the claims and counter-claims all end up being much of a muchness for Stephanie and all the other cancer patients struggling to make sense of it all.

You've been told you have cancer. You have had surgery to remove the tumor, and now you need chemotherapy. You also need time to absorb it all, but time, you are told, is what you don't have. Your oncologist mentions a new drug that, in combination with a couple of older ones, is showing promise. Let's call it "Elixir." As you leave the consulting room, the oncology nurse gives you a glossy pamphlet extolling the virtues of this new drug. The graphics are upbeat (rays of hope stream from clouds; doctors and patients smile warmly at each other), the text is perky and positive: "many people experience no side effects at all; although some might suffer hair loss, nausea, mouth sores. . . . Clinical trials have proven that 'Elixir'™ reduces risk of death by 23%." You wonder what that means. You would have a 23 percent greater chance of living forever? Or if you don't take it, you have a 77 percent chance of not dying. . . . Difficult enough to figure out the statistics without having to wonder if the therapy is being recommended to you because it really has shown promise or because its makers have sunk millions of dollars into its development and are trying to recoup some of that investment through a snazzy ad campaign.

Judy Erola, past president of the Pharmaceutical Manufacturers' Association of Canada, defends pharmaceutical advertising as education (CBC, 1997). "Is it marketing or is it education? There is no way a new product can receive any utilization in the world without appropriate education." It is a fine line.

A line that Paul Schubert thinks the pharmaceutical companies have long crossed. "When I was in hospital, my younger brother met some people who had a video of a doctor out of San Francisco talking about cancer and alternative methods. During the video she takes out the *American Medical Journal* and the *New England Journal of Medicine* and says, look how thick these journals are, but how much is actual articles on medicine? Very little compared to all the pages of advertisements from drug companies. So, her point was, who determines what goes in those magazines? . . . I don't know if I believe all this or not, but I think that there is something wrong."

It's a nasty scenario, the last thing you want to have to deal with when you are trying to choose what would be the best treatment for you.

As a cancer patient though, shouldn't you be reassured by the presence of the regulatory authorities with their mandate to protect the public good? Even if the drug companies are perhaps influencing research in some cases, as some experts claim, surely the authorities ensure that patients are still going to get the best treatment?

In Canada, the Health Protection Branch (HPB) is bound by criminal law to ensure that our food and drugs are safe. And it is charged with setting standards. However, its reputation has been tarnished by such recent events as the tainted-blood scandal in which its senior people were held accountable for lack of oversight and by accusations that it was suppressing the research findings of its own scientists as a result of industry pressure. The HPB is undergoing a reorganization that has some observers worried. Government cutbacks mean programs are disappearing and there are fewer resources. More research is being done by industry with the branch reviewing the results, rather than doing the research itself. Now corporations are paying 70 percent of the branch's budget through fees and, as the old adage has it, "Whoever pays the money, calls the shots." So it appears to be the case of the fox guarding the chicken coop. The move toward a self-regulating industry in health care is a dangerous road to be on. As one senior scientist says, "This direction is going to cost lives." The "Protection" in the Health Protection Branch is fading, and the public is not being told.

In late 1998, Health Canada (through the HPB) approved a chemotherapeutic drug called Xeloda in the treatment of advanced breast cancer. This approval was based on a clinical trial of 162 women across Canada, funded by the makers of the drug. The trial found that one in five women treated with the drug had a 50 percent or greater reduction in their tumors. One in five equals 20 percent, enough to gain regulatory approval. However, the trial also found that the drug did not extend the patients' lives.

As Gerald Lampe, a mesothelioma patient, wrote to the congressional hearings at the time of the closure of the IAT Clinic: "What does 'proven' mean when used to describe cancer therapy? When statistics 'prove' that a therapy is less than 20 to 30 percent effective in producing five-year survivals, how can this mean it is of proven value? Rather, does it not suggest that it is a proven failure?"

Xeloda is a chemotherapy that is being welcomed into the fold with an 80 percent failure rate. Apparently, it has received official sanction because it has been "properly" tested, not because it works. Semantics again: approved equals proven.

Meryle Berge is taking Xeloda for metastatic breast cancer. She was diagnosed in 1992, had the usual treatments, and was told that she was fine, to go away and live her life. She knew she wasn't fine, despite the assurances from her oncologist. When she asked for an MRI, her request was refused: MRIs are reserved for people who are in serious trouble, she was told. She had had Dr. Naessens's blood test, and it indicated that she was not clear of cancer, she was in serious trouble, but her oncologist was not convinced. She changed oncologists and had the MRI, which did indeed confirm metastatic disease. The cancer was in her bones now. "I do alternative therapies now," she said. "They are called clean food, clean air, and clean water. But you know, it's too late. The whole environment is poisoning us one way or another."

Her cancer is catching up: "Would you believe I used to be five foot seven? Look at me, I'm now five foot two. My rib cage is sitting on my hips." She gets around only with the help of a walker. She said, "I take Xeloda only as a crisis intervention. I'm taking it now. Maybe it's helping, I don't know. But the side effects are awful. It takes away who I am." Her short-term memory has been badly affected.

Yet this drug is approved, is considered "therapeutic." At the same time, biomedical treatments such as immuno-augmentative therapy and 714-X are not. Although never tested, they are effectively necklaced by the sobriquet "unproven."

Are these methods labeled "unproven" to protect the public? Yes, say the regulatory crew. Yes, say the pharmaceutical companies, which stand to make a whack of money on cornering the market for their drugs. Yes, say oncologists whose years in medical school and years of practice administering those drugs mostly close out the possibility of recognizing that they aren't doing the job. No, say the renegade doctors within the medical establishment who are recognizing that conventional approaches are not stopping the increase in cancer. No, say the researchers who, in their attempt to persuade the establishment at least to consider new directions in cancer treatment research, see the credibility of their work undermined by the label "unproven." No, say the critics of the cancer industry who see the approval of so many chemotherapies as simply a reflection of the power of business interests. And no, say the patients with a focus sharpened by the cancer still raging in their own bodies, despite the chemo or radiation they have endured.

11

The Scientific Method: A Hazard to Your Health?

Conventional—evidence-based—medicine relies on a rigid process of testing to determine the best treatments for a disease or medical condition. The process begins in the lab, moves through testing on animals, and culminates in what are essentially controlled experiments on people. Medical researchers don't use the term "experiments" much, preferring the foggy euphemism of "clinical trials." But no one could argue that, their label notwithstanding, they are experiments, pure and simple. The lawmakers are less semantically squeamish: "Medical progress is based on research which ultimately must rest in part on experimentation involving human subjects" (Medical Research Council, Canada, 1978).

Evidence-based medicine is both the means and the end in the scientific investigation of the causes and treatments of cancer; clinical trials are the culmination of the two, marrying research and practice in testing therapies in the real world of cancer care. Treatments developed through this approach are the only ones officially condoned by the medical mainstream. Observational studies, peer-review studies, and meta-analyses of studies already conducted complete the picture.

Regulatory agencies bestow the badge of acceptance on a cancer treatment, or the stamp of rejection, through clinical trials. Drugs, radiation therapy and dosages, combination therapies, kinds and extent of surgery, adjuvant therapies, hormone treatments, and vaccines—all must pass through the graduated sieves of the clinical trial process before being accepted into conventional primary cancer care.

At some point in your journey, and certainly not just as a last resort, you will encounter these litmus tests for everything from tamoxifen to toothpaste. In ads, when that professional-looking fellow wearing a white coat and stethoscope says, "Clinical trials have proven . . . ," we are programmed to accept the claim. Clinical trials say it works; it must be so. Who would deny science? It turns out, lots of folks. You will hear them say that clinical trials are misused, abused, misleading, biased, and fallible. You will also hear that clinical trials are the birthing fields for breakthroughs, the graveyards for snake oil, the watchdogs against quackery, and the conduit for the seeping of theory into practice.

Clinical trials come in four phases. Phase 1 trials, which can be used to study agents never before used on humans, are aimed at determining the safe and tolerable dosages of very new treatments. They are not geared to demonstrate whether the treatment is effective against the cancer. In fact, patients with a variety of cancers, size of tumor, and extent of metastasis are accepted into phase 1 trials; usually, though, they have all "failed therapies known to be of a benefit for their condition or have a tumor type for which no effective standard treatment regimen is currently known. . . . The initial patients entering a particular phase 1 trial receive a relatively low dose, anticipated to be tolerable based on prior animal studies or experience with agent(s) in other clinical settings. After several patients have received this dose and schedule, the next cohort of persons entering the trial will receive a predetermined larger dose of the agent(s). This process is continued until there is evidence of unacceptable toxicity at a particular dose level . . ." (Markman 1997, p. 12).

Phase 2 trials try to establish the antitumor effectiveness of a treatment or drug, administered according to a defined dose or schedule established by the phase 1 trial. Phase 3 trials compare a new treatment with the standard existing therapy. "The randomized phase 3 clinical trial is the ultimate test of the clinical utility of a new drug or strategy" (ibid., p. 12). Patients are assigned randomly to receive either the standard therapy, the new one, or, in some cases, a placebo. (Dr. Sue Aitken, medical oncologist, says that in twenty-five years of clinical medicine she has not encountered a chemotherapy, as opposed to hormone therapy trial, with a placebo as one of its arms. However, Dr. Bernard Fisher of the National Surgical Adjuvant Breast and Bowel Project (NSABP) talks of the placebo component in tamoxifen trials, and there are certainly placebo arms of vaccine trials.) A double-blind study means that neither the patient nor the doctor knows who is getting what. The assignment is mostly done by computer, often back at a central location geographically remote from where treatment is being administered. Informed consent of the patient going into a trial is particularly critical to phase 3 trials because of the random element. Patients must sign a document attesting to their understanding of their random assignment to one or other of the treatments in the trial. The purpose of phase 4 trials is to refine "the integration of the new treatment and determine its place in the primary treatment plan" (Altman and Sarg 1992, p. 66).

Thus, the scientific method fuels medical progress, slowly accumulating knowledge through controlled studies with stringent admittance criteria, set up so they can be replicated by other researchers. Gradually, over time, data accumulate and are analyzed and broken into statistics which then guide the next layer of investigation.

Dr. Robert Buckman says that clinical trials are "the only way knowledge advances . . . at present they are our only means of making true and credible progress against cancer" (1996, p. 322). There are those who disagree. Bill O'Neill, founder of the Canadian Cancer Research Group, argues that the whole premise of clinical trials is flawed: "Clinical trials of cancer therapies are based on the assumption that there are more similarities than dissimilarities in cancer so a trial can be set up on criteria related to these similarities. This is simply not the case. You might as well dump together someone with lupus, someone who has Parkinson's disease, and someone who grows onions and then set up a protocol to capture responses. All that we have learned from clinical trials is about things that don't work. . . . The process doesn't work. We need a new process to discern how this patient got his cancer, what is right and what is wrong with him, how is his disease different from another patient with the same diagnosis."

As usual in the world of cancer treatment, consensus on the subject is elusive.

Proponents of evidence-based medicine see its built-in checks and balances as the only way of protecting medical practices and patients from exploitation and costly, wasted efforts. They discount medical treatments or therapies driven by anecdotal or empirical evidence, arguing that proof of whether a treatment works must rely on statistical data. They say that accurate numbers cannot be drawn from anecdotal evidence because of the impurities of input, the unknown factors that can influence the outcomes. They posit that accurate statistics can be derived only from the controlled environment of clinical studies, the study of specific measurables, and the painstaking collection and analysis of the resulting data. Statistical success dictates acceptance of a treatment or therapy into the mainstream. But then, to your bafflement, you read something that seems to confound the central defense of medical science apologists altogether, that says most accepted treatment is *not* grounded solely in scientific data, not even by half.

A report of the Office of Technological Assessment states that 17 percent to 20 percent of conventional medical practices are based on scientifically validated evidence, which leaves 80 percent to 83 percent that are not (Beinfield and Beinfield 1997, p. 49). These are based on anecdotal evidence, the same foundation for which "unproven therapies" are condemned. It appears that the habit of some treatment practices overrides research findings that dispute the efficacy of those practices. "When clinical trials throw these habitual behaviors into question, rather than the behaviors adapting, studies are often functionally disregarded." In breast cancer treatment for example, "it was hypothesized that positive auxiliary nodes served as a predictor for the spread of the disease. When evidence indicated otherwise, only a few doctors altered their clinical behavior" (ibid.).

Then you hear what the critics have to say. They see the strict adherence to the scientific method as a straitjacket, constraining medical practices within criteria that are often irrelevant, easily manipulated, or misleading because of what they don't capture. They are convinced that the exclusive reliance on the scientific method to advance medical knowledge eliminates so much from the equation of healing that it could truly be retarding advances in some areas of cancer therapy. Taken to extremes, it also encourages the questionable practice—at least from the patients' point of view—of putting science (for the good of all) before the individual. They decry the reliance on statistics as a treatment's passport into the mainstream, pointing out how misleading the doublespeak of percentages can be: for example, an 18 percent success rate for a therapy really means that it fails 82 percent of the time. They argue that there is also proof in the pudding—if people thrive on a therapy, it should not be excluded from use because it has not been statistically verified. "Anecdotally" successful therapies are a product of the real world; therapies "proven" in clinical trials operate in the virtual world of aggregated data.

Lawrence Burton resisted randomized, double-blind trials because he believed it was unethical to have any patient *not* receive the treatment he so utterly believed in. Because of his faith in immuno-augmentative therapy, he felt that he would be condemning to death the group who did not receive it. The double-blind aspect he thought was just a cop-out, a way for doctors to avoid their responsibility to their patients: "Since you don't know whom you are handing death to, you are shielding yourself by saying, 'Oh, gee, it's double blind so I don't know who they are, so I'm not accountable.' My father wouldn't get involved with that at all" (Howard Burton, 1998 interview).

Between these two camps are those who agree that there has been progress made through evidence-based cancer research but at what cost? How often do clinical trials have to be conducted on, say, a chemotherapy drug, or a procedure such as bone-marrow transplantation, to prove that it doesn't work? they ask. They plead for the medical and regulatory community not necessarily to let go but at least to loosen the stranglehold of clinical trials on cancer treatment. They ask for a cessation of hostilities between the two factions, a recognition of the impact of unmeasurable elements in a patient's recovery, and a more humane and supportive environment for patient choice.

Suppose you come to that crucible when your doctor delivers the dreaded message, "There is nothing more we can do for you. Go home and put your affairs in order." And then he or she might add: "But there is a very new drug, it's in experimental stages still. It might help but I don't know. It has never been used for your type of cancer; it's being tested now. I could get you into the trial if you are interested."

You seem to have only two choices—give up, go home, and wait for the pain and dying, or go into the trial and take a long-shot with debilitating, "unproven" treatment. It's unlikely that your oncologist or radiologist would tell you at this point that there is another option, that you could seek treatment outside the mainstream—a treatment also "unproven," also a long-shot, but probably less damaging, possibly as effective, possibly more so. However, this is not perceived as a viable route because it is not part of the evidence-based process. So, you opt for the trial. As a participant, you now face a whole new tangle of perplexing issues.

First of all, the shiny, stainless-steel term "clinical trial" obscures the nub of the matter. These trials are not conducted on clinics; they are conducted *in* clinics and *on* people. Whether it's a dosage being established, or a new treatment being "tried" out against the old, you are the context of the trial. Your body and your cancer are the testing grounds, after all, so it can seem to be your trial, too. Especially when you read that prospective subjects for a trial are those patients "who fail other therapies."

Then you might ponder on how often the word "trial" is yoked with "and error." Trial and error is OK when you are doing a jigsaw puzzle, or maybe when you try out a new colour of nail polish. It's less palatable when it's your health, the quality of your life, and even your life itself at stake. But as environmentalist David Suzuki says, that is what the scientific method is all about. Science is the process of correcting past mistakes.

Finally, after doing some research, reading, surfing the Internet, and talking to doctors, it might dawn on you that clinical trials are not as precise as the term "clinical" suggests. They rarely arrive unequivocally at a finding; or they might do so for a year or two, but then another clinical trial refutes the first finding. And another. And so on. Despite the most rigid of criteria, unknowns creep in to shift the numbers. Or the numbers are calculated in a different manner, leading to different conclusions. That's the unfortunate way of statistics. Then a meta-analysis is done on all the clinical trial results to date and comes up with yet another conclusion.

As a prospective trial participant, you raise these issues. By doing so, you are revealing very cold feet. But clinical trials are sold hard to patients. Researchers need subjects upon which to conduct trials because the whole structure of evidence-based medicine rests on their availability. So, you are told that clinical trials are the gold standard of good medical investigation because the three "R"s—rigid criteria, replicable methods, and random assignment—impose the rigor of objectivity. You are assured that all clinical trials are reviewed by the hospital's or center's ethical committee to guard against unethical or dishonest practices; and you are assured that the random assignment of patients to one or other of the treatment protocols eliminates the possibility of biases in the outcomes of the trial. Results thus cannot be skewed by subjective or unknown influences.

That's the theory. And perhaps in theory it works most of the time. When you hear about the times it doesn't, these assurances sometimes ring hollow. For instance, with all these fail-safes built in, studies with similar criteria, methods, and random assignment should, theoretically, arrive at least within shouting distance of similar conclusions about a treatment or drug. Then you run smack up against the times they don't.

Example: A meta-analysis of non–small-cell lung cancer treatment results published in *The Lancet* in the summer of 1998 found that postoperative radiotherapy, an element of standard treatment in at least nine randomized trials over the years, not only did not increase survival of patients, it *increased* the risk of death by 21 percent (Stewart 1998).

Example: The American Academy of Dermatology and the Skin Cancer Foundation recommend the use of sunscreen to help reduce sunburn and skin cancer. These recommendations are based on studies. A multicenter case-control study concurrent with the recommendations to use sunscreen concludes that sunscreens do not protect against melanoma (GMDS 1996). Bristol University researchers published in the *British Medical Journal* in June 1999 that "there is evidence that the potential benefits of exposure to sunlight may outweigh the widely publicized adverse effects on the incidence of skin cancer." A Canadian dermatologist reports that some studies indicate that not only is sunlight a factor in skin cancer, it actually depresses the immune system.

Example: In the fall of 1988, the World Health Organization published the results of a ten-year study that concluded there was no link between second-hand smoke and lung cancer, or, in the words of the report, there was "a statistically non-significant positive association." However, a few months earlier the study's scientists had announced that their findings indicated a 16 to 17 percent risk of contracting lung cancer if you lived or worked with a smoker. These anomalies are from the same study.

Example: In clinical trials of tamoxifen as a preventive for breast cancer, the North American trial, the biggest cancer prevention trial ever in North America, found that tamoxifen cut the rate of breast cancer by nearly half over five years. It was announced that the study was cut short because of the enormous success of the drug and that it would be unethical, given the results, to continue giving a placebo to any of the women in the trial.

However, a six-year study by the Royal Marsden Hospital in London and a four-year study by the European Institute of Oncology in Milan found no difference in the incidence of breast cancer in women treated with tamoxifen or placebo (*Globe and Mail* 1998a). The Brits didn't approve of the early closing of the North American trials, claiming that we might be missing some important data downstream. We don't know the long-term results of such a drug on well women. Dr. Trevor Powles, leader of the British study, concluded: "I have grave concerns about the widespread use of [the drug] in healthy women" (Epstein 1998, p. 487). But Dr. Bernard Fisher, scientific director of the NSABP that conducted the tamoxifen prevention trial, said, "This is the first time in history that we have evidence that breast cancer cannot only be treated but also prevented."

When you look more closely at tamoxifen studies you find that the clinical trials have not cleared up the controversy surrounding the drug, but in fact have heightened it. You read that one of the reasons the North American study might have closed early is that doctors could not recruit enough women into the trials. It was a highly controversial undertaking, the first clinical trial in which a drug was tested on a healthy population. The goal had been to include 18,000 healthy women. Only 13,000 could be persuaded to take the drug. Many researchers were surprised and a bit miffed at the reluctance of well women to be guinea pigs. There was evidence that the drug had serious side effects, including uterine cancer and blood clots. At a conference on adjuvant cancer therapy, Dr. Bernard Fisher commented rather petulantly on the tamoxifen controversy: "We concluded that, when compared to placebo, the benefits from five years of tamoxifen, including a significant survival advantage, persisted through ten years of follow-up and that no additional advantage was obtained from continuing tamoxifen therapy for longer than five years. Finally, we found that the side effects from tamoxifen failed to preclude its use for the treatment of breast cancer. Moreover, in view of the benefits from tamoxifen, the findings with regard to the drug's undesirable side effects did not justify the recent political and media attack that created confusion in the minds of all women regarding the appropriateness of its use" (Fisher and Dignam 1997, p. 83). His comments are all the more confusing because he was talking about tamoxifen as a treatment for women who had breast cancer, and the really big controversy is about the drug being given as a preventive measure to healthy women who are at risk for getting the disease.

"All women" might be a little skeptical of Dr. Fisher's indignation in light of the fact that he was in charge of the National Surgical Adjuvant Breast and Bowel Project when it was revealed that doctors had been falsifying data to get their patients into the breast cancer treatment trials. The main culprit, Dr. Roger Poisson from St. Luc's Hospital in Montreal, claimed he had done it for the benefit of his patients because he knew they would get better treatment if they were in a trial.

You might be puzzled when you hear that Dr. Fisher had known of Dr. Poisson's actions for at least three years before they became public knowledge, but had neither reported the fraud nor re-evaluated the data to see how the trial results had been affected. It turns out that the National Cancer Institute and the National Institutes of Health had also been informed of Poisson's actions and had sat on the information for at least two years. Action was taken only when the press got hold of the story. Dr. Fisher, who was regarded as the Wayne Gretzky of breast cancer research (Hoy 1995) until this scandal sent him, however briefly, back to the minors, responded by asking the public to trust him. But the trust had been broken, by him, by Poisson, and by the regulatory agencies whose job it is to protect the public trust.

You might ask yourself, what is the point of those rigid criteria, if, when they are ignored, they don't affect the outcome of the trial, as was claimed by officials in charge of the study. Dr. Poisson called his altering of at least a hundred files "silly mistakes." You might think that surely scientists cannot have it both ways. Either the scientific method is followed to the letter (indeed, its credibility rests on its absolute accuracy of assessment and analysis) or it doesn't, in which case it is not good science. If it makes no difference whether someone fiddles with the data, the whole philosophy of the clinical trial approach is suspect, and you might conclude that clinical trials aren't such bedrock science after all.

Then, what are you to think when you hear that the problem with trials is not that their criteria are not stringent enough but that they are *too* stringent, so much so that they don't always apply to the general population? Yikes. But clinical trials are what guide direction in treatment, right? Yes. They are the basis for setting standards in practice for a particular kind and stage of cancer for everyone who has that cancer, right? Yes. Is there not a huge gap here, a leap of faith that must be taken by doctors and patients alike? For example, in breast cancer, a particular cocktail of chemotherapies worked well for women in a trial who exactly matched the criteria designed for that trial. Because of this success, the cocktail has become the gold standard for the general population of women with breast cancer. They would meet some of the major trial criteria (e.g., tumor size, whether there was metastasis, type of surgical procedure, whether they were pre- or postmenopausal), but the match would not be exact, nor would the same monitoring and controls as those used in the trial be in place. Patients still receive the treatment dictated by the trial, but will it work as well for them? Not always, says Dr. Sue Aitken. (Only about 5 percent of women being treated for breast cancer are in trials, not just because they don't want to be in one, but because they don't fit the criteria, their treating hospitals don't fit the criteria, or the infrastructure is not in place to support the tremendous amount of paperwork, testing, and follow-up.) So what gives? Well, the answer is "clinical trials give us clues, not certainties about how average women in day-to-day practice will respond to the treatments. And that's all we've got. Until a better method comes along, that's the way treatment findings inch forward," says Dr. Aitken.

You think you might go into the trial anyway. Whatever the overall trial results, you think you would still benefit personally and that in a trial you will receive leading-edge treatment based on the latest research. But this is not necessarily the case. It depends on the protocol to which you are randomly assigned—the current standard treatment or the new therapy being tested. You are assured that you will receive at least as beneficial a treatment as the standard therapy you would get in a non-trial setting. And then you remember that the "standard" treatment has achieved its status by virtue of previous clinical trials.

The question of bias keeps popping up. You are told that subjects are randomly assigned to the protocols within the trial so that neither the patient nor the trial administrators know who is getting what. How then could the results be skewed in favour of a particular outcome, you wonder, because you've found a survey of clinical trials published in a medical journal that says, "While 61 percent of drug studies in general reported results favourable to a new treatment, for studies supported by pharmaceutical companies the number soared to 89 percent. . . ." In other words, when the drug company is paying, nine out of ten times scientists find something positive to say, or say nothing at all.

This seems borne out by Dr. Nancy Olivieri's experience at the Hospital for Sick Children in Toronto. A blood researcher at the hospital, she agreed to test the drug deferiprone in clinical trials funded by the drug's manufacturer, Apotex. The drug was being used in the treatment of a rare and potentially fatal blood disorder called thalassemia. When she discovered that the drug was actually harming some of her patients, she reported her findings to Apotex. The company's response was to threaten legal action if she broke the confidentiality clause in her contract. She ignored the threat and told the patients of her findings. The ensuing scandal hit the front pages, drawing attention to the tarnish on the gold standard of clinical trials funded by vested interests.

Dr. Robert Rango is a clinical pharmacologist with the Therapeutics Initiative at the University of British Columbia, a provincially funded organization mandated to monitor how the pharmaceutical industry markets its clinical trials to doctors and the public. "There's all sorts of coercion," he says. "There's tremendous pressure from the industry because of all their deadlines. . . . They use doctors who can turn patients over. It's a factory mentality" (O'Hara, 1998).

The image is riveting. Under the circumstances, you might have serious misgivings about entering a clinical trial to be "turned over," roasting on the spit of science, basted by dishonesty and damage control.

Reliance on clinical trials can lead to some serious bending of statistics. Not a new concept certainly, but it is an unsavoury practice when statistics fudged through wishful thinking, avarice, duplicity, or just plain sloppiness are used as a foundation for launching or continuing a treatment that does not work or that actually does harm. This is a dangerous disservice not only to the people in a clinical trial but to all those patients and practitioners who rely on the accuracy of the trial to guide future cancer treatments.

Perhaps the biggest flaw critics see in clinical trials is that, despite all their apparent rigor, their outcomes are always suspect because of the very element they are incapable of assessing but also incapable of excluding. That is the human spirit. How can a clinical trial capture the impact of hope, of prayer, of the will to live? How can it measure the influence of compassion, of love? The protagonist of Richard Dooling's *Critical Care*, a savage and satirical novel about the current state of medical care, sums it up: "[The nurse] made a secret practice of compassion, even though it did not produce consistent, measurable results. If compassion, or kindness, or, God forbid, prayers produced any miracles, the results could not be duplicated; therefore, science had absolutely no use for them. Results might be interesting, provocative, sensational, miraculous, or astounding, but if they could not be duplicated by other scientists in a controlled setting, they were, by definition, useless to science and to the medical profession" (1992, p. 75).

The imponderables, the unquantifiables cannot be captured by criteria, nor do they lend themselves easily to statistical analysis, except to play havoc with any kind of rigid summations.

Clinical trials can give rise to conflicting conclusions, biased conclusions, conclusions made suspect by altered data, and conclusions skewed by the unmeasurable influence of the human spirit. Yet these same trials form the foundation for standard treatment protocols, the maps followed by cancer care practitioners, at least until a new map is drawn. A process with such apparent flaws seems shaky ground from which to criticize alternative approaches for their lack of scientifically proven efficacy.

Despite all the cracks in clinical trials, it still is usually not difficult to find participants. Cancer sufferers, desperate to try anything that might stem their disease, are often willing, indeed, plead to become trial fodder, even in phase 1 trials. What is not always made clear is that this phase of trial is concerned not so much with whether a treatment works, as with how much can be administered before it kills you. "[E]vidence from surveys of patients entering such studies reveals that the majority of those who participate in phase 1 trials consider therapeutic efficacy to be the aim of the programs" (Markman, 1997, p. 12).

The clear statement of the study's objective, to determine the level of "unacceptable toxicity at a particular dose level," makes sense to the scientist administering the study. After all, it is the goal of the exercise. But these words speak volumes in what they don't say, providing clinicians with the distance needed for objective observation, cloaking the searing reality of individual suffering. But you, as a subject in this experiment, can't fend off the pain through semantics. You jump into this uneasy mix of science and medicine as a person; you emerge as a calibration on a measuring stick of toxicity.

Braxton Colley's transmogrification from person to disease to number happened so fast his head spun. It was 1993, and he was feeling lousy again. His doctor diagnosed "walking pneumonia" and put him on antibiotics, to no effect. When he went back, his regular doctor was away. "You know, I've had this on and off for three years," he told the locum, who sent him for a series of tests. A pulmonary specialist drew fluid off the lung and a week later the results were back: cancer cells had been detected.

A biopsy confirmed the diagnosis: mesothelioma.

When Braxton and his wife, Hanna, spoke to the oncologist, they were told that chemotherapy and radiation had been found to be ineffective against mesothelioma. However, there was a clinical study under way right now for which Braxton was eligible. It was a chemotherapy trial. "If you want to go into the study, you have to sign up now because after today the study will be closed. There is no second chance to get in."

This is not an uncommon story. You hear often from cancer patients how they are told that they are lucky to be eligible for the trial, but that they must decide fast because the deadline for accepting new subjects is that day. I was told this by the researcher in charge of a breast cancer treatment trial in an Ottawa hospital. My diagnosis was less than a month old, my surgery had been done two weeks before, and so new was I to the cancer world I had no idea what a clinical trial was. But I was expected to make a decision that afternoon that could affect my life forever, not just the next ten months of treatment. The researcher thrust a sheaf of documents at me, urging me to sign up at once. These were the consent forms, pages and pages of dense legalese giving the medical profession permission to do anything and everything the lawyers could think up—with total immunity. I chose not to go that route.

My decision was easier than Braxton's; at first, he felt he had no choice at all. As presented by his doctor, it was the clinical trial or death. Added to the agony of trying to make such a decision was the nag that something wasn't making sense here. Hanna wanted him to seek a second opinion before making a commitment, because if chemotherapy didn't work on mesothelioma, why was he being urged to go into a clinical trial in which he would be given chemo? It turned out that the doctor did not like second opinions. It is hard to go against the full array of authority, especially when you've just been told that your husband has a terminal cancer and this might be his only chance.

The chemo he received in the trial very nearly killed him. "I couldn't eat, couldn't stand the smell of cooking. I lost sixty pounds."

Hanna said, "I just watched him getting smaller and smaller."

After several blood transfusions, a kidney failure, nausea, and hair loss, "I could not do it anymore. When I told the oncologist, he said, 'If you stop the treatment you can't go back on. You know, you will just go home and die.'"

The doctor's note to file in Braxton Colley's medical records confirms that he warned him that once he quit the treatment, he was out of the trial. It also confirms that the treatment was not doing a whit of good.

When Braxton asked just what the protocol was trying to prove, he says the answer was "to see how high a dose patients can withstand before it kills them." It was a phase 1 trial. Here was the bald truth of science staring Braxton in the face when he thought he was dealing with healing. The oncologist might have been talking about the FDA LD-50 lethal dose requirement of a clinical trial set-up, except that it wasn't mice they were testing the drug on now. Braxton quotes the oncologist again: "You know, four times your vital signs were so low, you couldn't take treatment. Weren't you a little amazed that each time on the last day, your signs suddenly got better so you could be given more chemo?"

The most basic of principles guiding the conduct of clinical trials as outlined in the Declaration of Helsinki as revised (1975) were falling like ninepins here: "Concern for the interests of the subject must always prevail over the interests of science and society. . . . Doctors should cease any investigation if the hazards are found to outweigh the potential benefits. . . .

In any research on human beings, each potential subject must be adequately informed of the aims, methods, anticipated benefits and potential hazards of the study and the discomfort it might entail" (Medical Research Council 1978, p. 62).

Braxton's case is not unique. A review of about 1,000 Food and Drug Administration spot-checks of the conduct of clinical trials between January 1996 and June 1999 found that 213 researchers failed to obtain proper consent from subjects, 364 failed to stick to their approved research plan, and 140 did not report adverse reactions from test drugs (Kaplan and Brownlee 1999, p. 34). In several cases, patients were not told of the standard treatments available but were persuaded to take experimental therapies.

Clinical trials had their beginnings in the early nineteenth century when Pierre Louis (1787–1872) first applied numbers to test therapies. He observed that a single case taught nothing, but if two groups of patients, randomly selected, underwent two different treatments, conclusions could be drawn through "arithmetic." His introduction of the scientific method into medicine was a mixed blessing. It provided practitioners with invaluable knowledge about treatments and patient response; but it launched medical research on a trajectory that pierces the very heart of healing. When medical researchers turn people into numbers, then medical practitioners are in danger of viewing them that way too.

Clinical trials are the crossroads at which science and healing collide. Braxton Colley, and many like him, at their most vulnerable, when they are least able to make clear-headed decisions, end up the victims of that collision. They are led there by some doctors who abandon the high ground of the precept "Do no harm" for the murky swamps of "good science." This is where the individual gets sacrificed on the stump of that often dangerously abused concept "the common good."

For the clinician whose paramount goal is to help, or at least not harm, individual patients in his or her care, the balance between human and scientific factors should not even be an issue. Clearly, the doctor's responsibility is to the individual patient.

For the scientist, however, clinical trials are a necessity for conducting medical research. By the early 1980s, it was estimated that chemotherapy saved approximately 3,000 patients a year under the age of thirty in the United States. The term "saved" is not defined, but presumably it means extending the patient's life by more than five years. One scientist concluded that these numbers represented "very real gains" and were a fitting memorial to the many thousands of patients who took part in the early trials of various forms of chemotherapy to get there (Patterson 1987, p. 197).

But the scientist still has a responsibility to weigh the human costs against the scientific gains. Of all the branches of science, progress in medical science is rightly hampered by such considerations. You can't just take a population of human beings and experiment with them the way scientists can take a group of rats or monkeys or birds. When a proposal was made to do just that, using experimental AIDS drugs on populations in developing countries, there was such an outcry that the suggestion was quickly abandoned. However, you could understand why such an approach would appeal to the scientist. The assumption is that the people involved in the testing of the drugs were doomed anyway, so they might as well be used to benefit future generations.

And, of course, such human testing *has* been done, but without publicity and, apparently, without "informed consent" from the people on whom the drug is being tested. The LSD experiments in Kingston, Ontario, at the federal Prison for Women in the early 1960s, are one example. A lawsuit filed by one of those inmates in July 1998 brought this response from the man who had been head of psychiatry at the time and who had approved the tests: "It was good research back then. It's still good science," he said. "That's why we did it, to see what would go on." He has no plans to offer any apologies. "That's the government's problem, not mine," he said. "To hell with it" (*Ottawa Citizen*, 1998a). In another interview, the retired psychiatrist, now eighty-four, suddenly clammed up, and wouldn't say anything more to the interviewer except, "I'm going fishing." Which is what he was doing when he was practicing his "good science."

It is not surprising that many patients resist being turned into fodder for the voracious maw of science and instead set out on a route that takes them to places such as the IAT Clinic, where they retain their status as persons and find emotional support not available "back home."

That is what Braxton Colley did. When he finally could not stand the experimental chemotherapy any longer, he made another choice, one that he hadn't realized was there for him when the clinical trial was first proposed. He opted for the gentler terrain of an empirical-based alternative treatment— immuno-augmentative therapy. Ironically, there was one similarity between the two therapies; they are both "unproven." Yet the chemo, which was doing no good and making Braxton so desperately ill, is supported by the establishment because it was part of a clinical trial, whereas the immuno-augmentative therapy, which seems to have brought his cancer under control for the last six years and given him back his life, is still beyond the pale. At the IAT Clinic, it didn't seem to be such a no-win situation: a toss-up which would get you first—the cancer or the treatment.

The scientific method of advancing knowledge has the modern world in such thrall it seems churlish to question its role in medicine. Clinical trials have pointed the way to the apparent benefits of adjuvant therapy in the treatment of breast cancer, and of chemotherapy in childhood leukemia. A cynic might ask whether these are the mistakes that future scientists must correct, or genuine breakthroughs. But in other areas of medicine, science has accomplished so much—anaesthesia, antibiotics, pain relief, less invasive diagnostic techniques, the near eradication of such scourges as smallpox, cholera, polio, and syphilis. And the marriage of medicine and technology has produced the whole transplant industry—hearts, lungs, livers, kidneys, pancreas. Severed limbs are sewn back on; hips are replaced; breasts are rebuilt; there are skin grafts for burn victims, pacemakers for faulty hearts, new faces for a variety of reasons—cosmetic, disguise, and reconstruction. There are medicines that keep schizophrenics on an even keel, drugs to keep depression at bay. There are almost-invisible digital hearing aids that suppress peripheral noise. There is laser surgery to improve eyesight, re-attach retinas, destroy skin cancer cells, remove moles, or fix knee cartilage. "Our capacity to fix, repair, replace and cure seems to be limitless," says Dr. William Molloy in his book *Vital Choices: Life, Death and the Health Care Crisis* (1993, p. 15).

Not quite. Many cancers elude this round-up of successes, slinking along beyond the reach of medical science, pulling people down at will. It is cruel and deceitful to claim that chemotherapy and radiation can cure most cancers. (Childhood leukemias and Hodgkin's disease are the exceptions, and those often at a huge cost to the patient's later health.) At best, these difficult treatments control disease for a while, often sacrificing quality of life for a few additional weeks or months; at worst they kill the patient. Yet cancer patients are still told, despite proof to the contrary, that the only route to successful treatment is scientific testing through clinical trials which "prove" the accepted methods. "Unorthodox cancer treatments should be avoided because they don't work and could be dangerous," says David Drum in his 1998 book, *Making the Chemotherapy Decision*: "Some happy day . . . your chemotherapy treatments may be complete. At that time, with a clean bill of health, you'll be ready to move on with your life" (p. 236). Tell that to Braxton Colley.

Patients must be aware—must be made aware—that the primary objective of a clinical trial has nothing to do with their individual health, and everything to do with the therapy being tested; as a participant you are a tool in an experimental process, which, it is hoped, will eventually benefit someone. The random assignment of patients to the various arms of a trial underscores the general objectives, which have less to do with people than with science. Not to put too fine a point on it: "Until we know the best and definitive treatment of cancer, every patient will be a guinea-pig" (Buckman 1996, p. 322). This is a hard concept for a sick pig to grasp.

However, even as a guinea pig, you have rights. You have the right to assume that the treatment you receive in a trial at least has the possibility of helping you. You have the right to expect that treatment dosages alone aren't going to kill you. You have the right to expect that the trial results will be honest. *And you have the right to know that there are viable alternatives to clinical trials.*

12

The Art of Healing versus the Science of Medicine

Many people are turning away from conventional treatment not only because of the therapy itself but also because of how it is delivered. Science, technology, and the narrowing focus of medical specialties have shorn treatment to a razor-sharp focus on the cell, the disease, the tumor. This is good science but not good medicine, say more and more physicians. Dr. Ruth Ann Barron, a homeopathic doctor from Toronto, says, "You know why a place like IAT works for so many patients? Because it supports the patient the way conventional medicine used to, before the advent of the specialist."

Ross Pelton writes in his preface to *Alternatives in Cancer Therapy*: "I believe one of the most important factors in cancer treatment is recognizing the needs and experience of our patients. . . . Patients need to know that there is hope for recovery and that the treatments they receive will not make death appear preferable to more suffering. One of the most important insights the medical establishment could learn from alternative therapists is the value of a patient-centered approach" (Pelton and Overholser 1994, p. 8).

This philosophy may be the main feature that attracts people to alternative therapies and makes believers out of patients. These practitioners listen, empathize, and, in some form, say, "I'll do the very best I can to make you better." Against the backdrop of science, in the world of conventional treatment, doctors link their message to the statistics; with metastatic cancer, this means saying, in effect, "You don't have a hope." The will to live is a powerful thing, especially when it is yoked with the will of a healer to help you live.

For a variety of reasons, alternative cancer centers provide the infrastructure of care for the whole person. Sometimes it's because they don't have the financial resources to streamline and "improve" their systems, as at the IAT Clinic in the Bahamas, where patients have built their own infrastructure. Sometimes there is a conscious focus on the whole person, as at Oasis, where the spiritual and emotional aspects of illness are recognized as being as influential as the physical elements.

Sound familiar? The term "patient-centered medical care" is floating through the literature now as if it were a brand-new concept. And that is a *scary* thought. If medical care is *not* focused on the patient, just what is it focused on? A generation or two ago, we had patient-centered care: people went to their family physicians for everything. These doctors knew their patients from birth to death. They had the context of the person's life, they had the broad picture in which the cancer appeared. That family doctor was indeed a "family" doctor. He or she (usually "he") knew the parents and often the grandparents of the patient; knew the children; knew the house they lived in, where they worked, probably had attended at their birth, and would probably attend at their death. When cancer was discovered in a person's body, it was not just the body these doctors treated, but the whole person. The concept of GP as traffic cop had not taken hold yet.

Now, patients are quickly referred to specialists—specialists in diseases and specific parts of the body. The whole is not even the sum of its parts. This development has led to highly fragmented medical service at big treatment centers. It would be more convenient for everyone if the patient's body could be divided up among appointments: send the arm with its veins to the lab for blood tests, the breast to a surgeon for a biopsy, the chest to radiology for X-ray. . . .

The most obvious arrangements—such as grouping a cancer patient's appointments to save travel time or giving patients the results of tests within a day or two to reduce the stress of waiting—are still considered highly innovative in the few places such practices have been introduced. After decades of prodding, a few cancer-treatment facilities have gathered additional resources, such as psychotherapy and support groups for cancer patients, but these still remain way down on the priority list. "The modern hospital often forgets the person and treats the disease. The object of the treatment is to shrink the cancer, put the disease in remission or remove the growth. In spite of wonderful medical successes, more and more we feel the emptiness, humiliation and frustration of this experience. . . . The modern hospital does not provide *health* care but *sickness* care ..." (Molloy 1993, p. 254; emphasis in original). In the management of cancer care, the patient often seems to come last in the practical priorities, an attitude encouraged by the swing away from personal to technological care, from healing to medicine.

"You can't go through the medical world these days without a navigator at your side," Dr. Sue Aitken says. "I hate to say it but it's true." Cancer patients need someone to ensure that things happen, to follow up, to make the connections between the various islands of specialties, to coordinate care. They need one access point into the system. Dr. Aitken says that an Ontario Breast Screening Program pilot project in Hamilton, Ontario, has produced data that Britain and Europe have known for years, that "when screening and assessment are tightly linked, when patients and families are guided through the system, treatments are more timely. . . . Patients and their families must have access to information and consultation at all times."

This does not seem to be an earth-shattering discovery, but it is a wake-up call for a system that has shifted its focus from patients to process. In part, the skewing of priorities may spring out of the testing ground of residency training, where the gruelling demands on fledgling doctors sometimes burn out the humanity that led them to choose to be doctors in the first place. "Although the relationship with the patient is central to medicine, it may be the most neglected area of learning in residency training. . . . personal discomfort, fatigue, time pressures, and team conflicts often erode this relationship until residents become numb to the emotional needs of patients. This increased emotional buffering . . . is a form of denial that precludes a unique possibility for supervised learning and for exploration of painful issues in care. Although technical medical care may be provided, no holistic healing takes place" (Peterkin 1998, p. 76). It is a pattern that, established at residency stage, seems to stay with many doctors throughout their careers.

Such attitudes, absorbed by doctors through a fog of exhaustion in their residency period, are now enhanced by the science of medicine. Burgeoning technology, the plethora of new drugs, the emphasis on clinical trials and the numbers approach to medicine—all have widened the gap between doctor and patient. It is a rent in the fabric of human contact that a few years ago was at the heart of health care. It is an irony that success in the "hard" tools of medicine—knowledge and technical progress—appears to be negated by failure in the "soft" skills of compassion and communication.

In December 1991, a panel of physicians in Toronto reported that "doctors on average interrupt their patients within 18 seconds of beginning to be told the presenting problem. Moreover, 54 percent of patient complaints and 45 percent of patient concerns are never discussed" (Valerie Mindel, quoted in Molloy 1993, p. 23). If this is the state of the nation in a standard consultation about, say, flu symptoms or backache, imagine how much worse the communication can become when the consultation is about a cancer diagnosis. Dr. Robert Buckman says he hopes that people will stop cringing over the word "cancer." Well, they won't, not until there is more certainty about the outcome of treatments. So when a person is told that she has cancer, whatever the kind, whether it be totally curable skin cancer or totally incurable stage 4 pancreatic cancer, she is going to do more than cringe. It's not going to help the individual patient to be told that if she looks at cancer as a group of chronic diseases, then "we [the medical profession and researchers] are not doing so badly" (Buckman, quoted in *Ottawa Citizen*, February 8, 1999a). The semantics here mean diddly-squat to the new cancer patient. Only one message is as clear as a shard of glass: You have cancer.

Patients are trying to understand through a sieve of stress and fear what the doctor is telling them. Dr. Buckman writes about how research into what causes cancer can miss the mark. "If you ask the 'wrong' questions, not only will you miss the right answer, you might actually come to the wrong conclusion" (1996, p. 31). Transfer this scenario to a consultation between a physician and a patient (or a patient's family) and imagine the possibilities for "wrong conclusions," since mostly the patient *doesn't* know the right questions to ask. It has to be the physician's responsibility to ensure that the "right answers" are given anyway, that information is provided as clearly and simply as possible, and as many times as necessary.

It is true that adequate communication is becoming increasingly difficult for physicians because of time constraints, heavy case loads, and the fact that patients are asking more detailed questions, are coming armed with more information (or misinformation), and—especially younger patients—are determined to have input into the decisions regarding their treatment. Such challenges notwithstanding, it is still not the patients' responsibility to coax doctors into doing their jobs properly. Patients have enough to deal with without having to play mind games with those doctors who forget that their job is to help *people*.

Edwina Smith met such a doctor when she sought a second opinion about whether to have a bone-marrow transplant. When she asked if he had ever treated her kind of cancer before, he was enraged. Edwina says, "I think he thought I was questioning his credibility, but frankly I was the one standing there with the rare cancer. . . . It was one of the worst encounters I've ever had in my life with anyone, let alone a physician. . . . I cried all the way home."

At the time, bone-marrow transplants were a new treatment for solid tumors—not even through clinical trials yet. "I was very frightened . . . of basically shutting down my life and then dying before I got any life back, like, life as in living. There were huge risks, and I was very scared," she says quietly.

What she did not need, on top of the disease, the treatment she had already endured, and the fear, was a doctor who bullied and patronized her. Doctors have a responsibility to do better. Patients should not have to bear the brunt of a doctor's lack of social or communication skills.

It is an old, old lesson, though one apparently forgotten in the brave new world of technology and specialization. As Hippocrates wrote: "Some patients, though conscious that their condition is perilous, recover their health simply through their contentment with the goodness of the physician" (Nuland 1995, p. 17).

Some are attempting to relearn this lesson. Dr. Aitken says that medical schools are making an effort to ensure that students meet real people sooner in their training. And "communication skills" are now included in the curriculum. The result should be more compassionate doctors. However, Aitken says, "the increasing complexity of medicine today demands that you rely on technology instead of what used to be called clinical sense." The ability to observe, listen, examine, and identify possible disease processes is being replaced by reliance on technology. And this is exactly what drove one Canadian nurse out of her profession: "I knew what all the bells and whistles on all the machines meant, but if you asked me I often wouldn't know if the patient hooked up to those machines was a man or woman."

Patients do better when they can stay human. "Since technology deprives me of the intimacy of my illness, makes it not mine but something that belongs to science, I wish my doctor could somehow repersonalize it for me. It would be more satisfying to me, it would allow me to feel that I *owned* my illness, if my urologist were to say, 'You know, you've worked this prostate of yours pretty hard. It looks like a worn-out baseball.'" (Broyard 1992, p. 47).

It is a tightrope doctors must walk. You see it in patients' medical records. The juxtaposition of the medical records in the filing cabinets, and the patients in the treatment rooms is a searing reminder of the dichotomy doctors face daily.

In her medical file, a woman with breast cancer has been deconstructed into body parts. Her pathology report reads as follows:

> Specimen A . . . consists of fatty tissue. . . . Towards one side it contains a rocky hard, stellate-shaped, whitish tumor mass measuring 1.8 × 1.5 × 1.5 cm. Frozen section diagnosis: carcinoma.

> Specimen B . . . consists of breast weighing 980 grams and measuring 25.0 × 22.0 × 4.5 cm. The nipple is everted and grossly normal . . . the skin is light tan . . . and there are no gross abnormalities.

Except one. It is no longer attached to her body.

Some doctors can't make the switch from parts to person. The real woman, the whole woman, the sum total of those parts, frightened and bruised in both body and spirit, sits in the doctor's office looking for reassurance, for wisdom, for a way out. However, the doctor looks up from her medical file and sees not a whole person but "breast cancer." Left breast, right breast, the details don't seem to matter that much, judging from the sloppiness of entries in some medical files. In one, a doctor has written: "Diafinography is unremarkable except that it does show three masses on the right breast. . . ." Someone has stroked out "right" and written in the margin "LEFT!" underlined twice. Later in this same report: "As far as the opposite cancer effected right breast, she has made a

decision to go conservative and I am not objectionable at all."
"She" might disagree. This same doctor is irritated that his
patient is going to try an alternative therapy: "I think this is a
rather foolhardy undertaking which indicates possibly a
degree of worrisomeness on the part of this patient. Obviously
she is not content to the care that she has received because she
is now going for further . . . experimental, nonproven, non-
tested, no peer reviewed therapy." Her "worrisomeness"
might be well-founded, given that this doctor can't seem to
remember which breast her cancer is in. Another file I read the
same morning had the same mistake: "official diagnosis:
extensive, multifocal infiltrating and intraductal carcinoma
of the left breast." Apparently not. Again, a firm hand has
changed "left" to "right."

Following a biopsy, Berris Pantaluk was told that she had
breast cancer, with ten nodes positive (cancerous lymph nodes
in her arm pit, indicating that the cancer was on the move
from its original site). The oncologist broke the news: "I give
you a very poor prognosis even with chemo and radiation.
You have maybe a 30 percent chance for recovery. I'll take you
to the nurse." Berris says, he then stood up, walked to the
door, and called the nurse to get a booklet on chemo. "He did
not say, 'Do you have any questions?' He didn't say anything
supportive at all."

Her husband was with her to hear the news: "We couldn't
speak. We were devastated. The surgeon had said 'You're
going to be fine.' We were expecting the same support from
the oncologist, but it wasn't there."

Berris's husband called the oncologist: "I don't understand
why you give my wife so little chance to live." The oncologist's
response? "You'd better start to face the hard cold facts. Any
more questions?"

This doctor may be the best technician in the world, may be the finest practitioner of medicine, but he's no healer. Of a list of rules for residents on how to deliver bad news (Peterkin 1998, pp. 79–80), this fellow broke all but one.

- "Bad news is best delivered when you have time for the patient." He appeared to have about a minute and a half before ushering them out to the nurse.
- "Watch patients for all-important non-verbal cues as to how they are listening to you. Be prepared for strong emotions and acknowledge them." He didn't appear to notice Berris's tears, her husband's stunned silence.
- "Give patients the chance to be prepared for what you say." He gave no warning.
- "Patients must be given time to express their fears and worries." Nope, again.

The one rule he followed? "Straightforwardness and lack of prevarication are essential."

In their search for a medical team to treat Earl's metastatic cancer, Earl and Leslye Kruger interviewed doctors from several hospitals. They were advised to see a surgeon—"the best in the city," they were told by another doctor. Earl said, "We checked him out. He was top drawer as a surgeon, bottom of the heap in humanity." Leslye was more succinct. "He was a prick."

When he saw Earl's records, he told them, "This is a complicated case, I'll get back to you." Two weeks went by. Finally the Krugers called for an appointment. The surgeon didn't have time but would talk to Earl by phone. They set up a time and sent the surgeon some questions beforehand. He did not call back at the appointed time. They called his secretary to set up another telephone appointment. It happened again. He did not call back. A third appointment was set up. This time the doctor did call . . . three hours after the agreed time.

"You asked me a million questions," he said. "I don't have the answers to any of them."

Leslye says dryly, "These were not hard questions. For example: Were there clear margins on the tumors? Will Earl need physiotherapy after his operation?"

Good doctor? Maybe. Healer? No. Three days later, Earl and Leslye pulled all Earl's medical records and went to another hospital.

"[W]hile technology has provided dramatic cures and techniques, it has also separated us from human feelings and made it harder for health professionals to feel compassion or concern for their patients. Many doctors, blinded by the awesome power of the technology they use, have lost touch with the emotional needs of their patients" (Molloy 1993, p. 23).

This might be a clue to one of the most puzzling questions in cancer treatment: Why do some people recover from a supposedly terminal cancer while others, with the apparent same diagnosis, grade, and stage of the disease, die? Clearly, no one knows, although the theories are legion. Some medical researchers say it has to do with genes, or cells, or enzymes. Some environmental scientists say it depends on whose immune system is strong enough to withstand the toxicity of our planet. Other epidemiologists, such as those who claimed that a cluster of five breast cancers in a population of fifty employees working on one floor of a building in Hamilton happened by chance, still deny a connection between environmental contaminants and cancer. Statisticians believe the numbers, whatever they say, and work at explanations when the numbers collide. Doctors believe it is the brand of medicine they practice that makes the difference, whether it be chemotherapy or coffee enemas. Some cancer patients believe that their life or death is absolutely in God's hands; others credit fate, karma, or random luck.

Many cancer patients believe their survival has to do with attitude, with support systems, or with having a goal to keep them alive. But there are few who deny the importance of hope and of faith in their chosen "healer."

Healers have been featured players down through the ages and in every culture—shamans, witches, elders, priests, holy men . . . and doctors. The power of a healer is a mystery that defies science. So science scoffs and denies the power it cannot decipher. In 1763, the Scottish surgeon John Bell denounced shamans whom he saw in action in southern Siberia as "a parcel of jugglers, who impose on the ignorant and credulous vulgar." In his history of medicine, Porter writes: "Such a reaction is arrogantly ethnocentric: although shamans perform magical acts, including deliberate deceptions, they are neither fakes or mad. Common in native American culture as well as Asia, the shaman combined the roles of healer, sorcerer, seer, educator and priest, and was believed to possess god-given powers to heal the sick" (Porter 1997a, p. 32). Healers have had a hard time of it through the ages. Jesus, the quintessential healer, was nailed to the cross; witches and midwives were burned or drowned; physicians ahead of their time in medical knowledge and practice were often vilified in their lifetime.

Does a healer's power come from a divine source, is it a practical skill, or does it lie only in the faith of the healed? When the healing works, for the afflicted, does it matter? "It comes as no earth-shaking revelation that the confidence of the patient in his physician is one of the cardinal factors in the art of healing" (Nuland 1995, p. 17).

Lawrence Burton was not a doctor, but for many he was certainly a healer. Charlotte Gerson is not a doctor, but for the woman in the front row of the presentation on the tour of the

Mexican clinics, she is a healer. According to the U.S. regulatory agencies, Burzynski is a fraud and a criminal; in the eyes of his patients, he is a healer. Dr. Naessens is not a medical doctor; he has never practiced medicine. But for the people whose cancer has been checked by his therapy, 714-X, he is a healer.

Healers, of course, can be found in the clinics, corridors, and consultation rooms of conventional cancer treatment too. At an educational forum on breast cancer in Pembroke, Ontario, Dr. Sue Aitken, not only an oncologist but until her retirement in the summer of 1999 head of the Ontario Breast Screening Program, gave a presentation on the program. She had slides and charts and talked of thirty cancers out of a thousand being detected in this early warning system. She papered the room with statistics and extolled a system within the conventional medical model. Her presentation was practiced, seamless, and positive. Early detection plus conventional interventions of surgery, chemotherapy, and/or radiation were the cornerstones of success in beating breast cancer.

Following the formal part of her talk, she took questions from the floor, and in that instant, when she stopped speaking to an audience and began to communicate with individuals, her true calling shone through. She is a healer. She spoke directly to each questioner; she did not prevaricate, pontificate, or lecture. She did not spout the party line for any form of cancer therapy but offered considered and thoughtful advice on natural therapies, on conventional therapies, on attitudes, and on patient-doctor relationships. She spoke from the heart to the heart. After question period, a line of women formed to speak to her, and she had time for each one; she listened, her eyes studying their faces; she touched a hand, examined a proffered arm bloated with lymphodema, hugged women whose tears told of a recent diagnosis or recurrence.

And she gave to each one something more precious than medical advice: she gave them her undivided attention in a crowded, noisy room; she gave them humor and intelligence and the sum of her experience; most valuable of all, she gave them hope. And therein lies the difference. Communications courses by the peck will not turn a technician into a healer. Patients see through the lip-service. There must be the genuine connection, a shared recognition of the human condition.

Dr. Aitken and others like her transcend the wretched skirmishes and posturing of the medical wars in which so many cancer patients find themselves enmeshed. They don't succumb to science; they have long ago shed their blinkers, if, indeed, they ever had them. Dr. Aitken became an oncologist because of "a good experience and a less than stellar one: the combination made me into an oncologist." She did her internship through Women's College Hospital at Toronto's Princess Margaret Hospital in the 1970s. "For two months I saw radiologists, medical oncologists, and physicians all treating each other as human beings in the context of a wealth of medical challenge." But then her young husband developed colon cancer and she experienced the medical system from the other side, a much darker side. "I saw first hand then how it didn't work; I saw how he was treated, how I was treated as his spouse, even though I was a doctor. I saw what he wasn't told, I saw how he was told things, I saw the lack of communication with him and me. And I knew there had to be a better way."

Dr. Aitken was my oncologist. She was the one who told me after my breast cancer diagnosis and surgery, "We have one kick at the can so we have to kick it hard." And proceeded to kick with me every step of the way. She was forthright and honest, and not once did she ever patronize, resort to technobabble, or use the crushing demands on her time as an excuse not to be there for me when I needed more than information on blood counts and anti-nausea drugs. Years later, when I thanked her for everything she had done during those dark days of chemotherapy and fear, she would not take the credit. She said, "We made a good team."

Doctors like Sue Aitken never lose sight of the person inside the disease. They don't protect themselves by closing off to the pain and fear of their patients; they somehow reach through their own feelings; they make contact. They truly communicate, not because they have taken courses in how to talk to patients or acquire a perfect bedside manner. It is much deeper and more visceral than that. They appear to respond instinctively to a patient's need for more than physical doctoring. They are practiced in the ways of the heart and the mind as well as the body. They know how to bring a patient through the fear and doubt, always providing a route to hope. Obviously, they cannot heal every patient, "but [a person's] illness may be eased by the way the doctor responds to him— and in responding to him the doctor may save himself. . . . It may be necessary to give up some of his authority in exchange for his humanity, but as the old family doctors knew, this is not a bad bargain" (Broyard 1992, p. 57).

Dr. Robert Buckman describes that something extra in all good consultations that cannot be reduced to one simple element. He calls it a chemistry or perhaps an alchemy which can result when the healer's wish to help the patient combines with the patient's wish to get well. Woolly Setteducato's surgeon was a healer, not just because he was skilled in the techniques of his profession. He had great hands that could guide a scalpel through the human body and sew the wound back up with a minimum of mess. He also had a great heart, and the intelligence to recognize the power of non-scientific elements in Woolly's recovery against all odds, the power of the will to live.

These are the doctors to look for. If you come to that point when you must hear the message that your cancer is winning, you'll want to hear it from a doctor who understands that it is not a death sentence.

There are ways of delivering the tough message without destroying hope. The doctors who do this are the ones who recognize that they are not God, that the future is unpredictable, that one can never be certain of an outcome, and that therefore there is always room for hope. A good doctor can recognize that, from his or her vantage point (medical experience and education), the condition might appear hopeless, but not the person. How does a doctor deliver this message? There is a fear of holding out false hope—although most patients would say there is no such thing, there is only good hope. People can hold two views of their situation: they can understand that their situation is looking hopeless, but they themselves can be hopeful of a different outcome. This is not denial. This is an integral part of the treatment. The Hope Foundation at the University of Edmonton, Alberta, has done studies indicating that if patients have no hope, they don't participate in their treatment. It is the crux of any treatment. Without hope, "they won't even get out of bed in the morning."

The foundation's research suggests that to "access" hope, you must have a trusting relationship with your doctor. If your doctor reaches the point where he or she must honestly say, "There is nothing more we can do," optimism dies because optimism stems from predicting the future based on the past. But if your doctor adds, "Go home and put your affairs in order. No, there is nothing else out there for you, so forget it," hope dies too, the belief that because the future is uncertain, anything can happen. That is perhaps one of the main differences between a technician who practices medicine and a doctor who practices healing: the ability to convey hope. Or the skill not to destroy it.

In the current climate of cancer treatment, it seems to many patients that the healers are losing out to the technicians. These are the doctors who, for whatever reason, take cover in the thickets of technology, losing sight of the individual patient and focusing on the parts, not the sum of a person, on a disease, but not the humanity it is devouring. In fact, Peterkin lists "identification of patients by body part, disease, or room number" as one of the danger signals of burnout for residents (1998, p. 77). The science of medicine thrives in the shade of technology's thickets. The art of healing doesn't.

In an address to the graduating class at the University of Toronto's Faculty of Medicine, the Nobel Prize–winning chemist John Polanyi cautioned against replacing compassion with science: "In science the crucial balance is between seeing things whole and seeing them in part. Nature deals in forests, scientists seldom even in trees. . . . By putting on blinkers and seeing only a part of a complex phenomenon we reveal connections previously hidden from view. These linkages are the stuff of science. But in the process of delving for hidden patterns the larger pattern called a forest can be lost to view. Then the strength of science, which lies in its sharp but narrow focus, becomes its weakness. . . . The question of balance between the picture and its details is as central to your profession as it is to mine. The medical arts in their eagerness to be accepted as science have striven for precision. You are awash at this moment in an ocean of measurables. This is valuable . . . so long as one is reminded—for example, by looking in the mirror—that the patient is not an equation" (reprinted in the *Ottawa Citizen*, July 16, 1998c).

Sometimes doctors are put back in touch with the true calling of medicine through a particular patient, one who holds up that mirror. Woolly Setteducato was such a patient. He either attracted the best doctors, or transformed them into good doctors with his humor and zest for life. He and his wife, Ida, sat waiting for the doctor, who was late for the appointment. When he came into the examination room, Woolly greeted him with a grin and a hearty handshake. "We won't take up your time, doctor. I'll just take your temperature, listen to your heart, and you'll be on your way." By switching persona, Woolly was unconsciously reminding the doctor of their shared humanity, and that, in a nanosecond, the doctor could be the patient, finding himself at the wrong end of the scalpel or stethoscope.

Dr. Marc Flitter, a neurosurgeon, describes a brain surgery that went wrong:

> Send this for frozen section. Label it brain tumor. . . . The metallic voice of the pathologist confirmed the diagnosis on the speaker phone, dispassionately announcing in deadly alliteration, "anaplastic astrocytoma." But the diagnosis was no longer the problem. There was no clot that I could see and yet the tissue kept coming, extruding like lava without apparent end. . . . By then it was too late. Underneath those paddies lay a quiet pool of ruin and devastation that could not be undone. There was no need to wait until the morning to assess the damage. The patient would not survive. I had seen this before, in my own cases and those of my colleagues and professors.

Then, almost unannounced—I certainly hadn't sent for her—Judith returned to the room. It wasn't just a small opening in sterile drapes through which brain tissue had herniated that was my charge. A human being lay there, now irreversibly lost. She was not bionic woman, to be made good as new with a prosthesis and rehabilitation. She was mother and wife undone, as removed from the world of her family as if she had died last year and had been buried back in Ohio. (1997, pp. 23–25).

Surely this is what doctors try to protect themselves from. By focusing on nothing but that incision draped in sterility, they can trick themselves into not seeing that beneath their scalpel lies a human being. They must keep their mind free of the clutter of another's life—the pain, fear, and suffering that have brought the person to the surgical table in the first place—for two reasons. First, to do what they are trained to do, with skill and certainty, allowing no distractions to blur their focus: "I had been conditioned during my medical training not to react viscerally to a patient's pain and suffering. Otherwise, my judgment would be impaired and my effectiveness limited in responding to the needs of my patients" (Groopman 1997, p. 160). And second, to avoid the unnerving experience of staring straight into the eye of their own mortality.

The surgeon is, at least for the moment, on the right end of the scalpel; the oncologist, at the plunger end of the chemo needle. For the moment. Perhaps doctors cloak themselves in science and technical terms to ward off the realization that the next skull cracked open to reveal an inoperable tumor could be their own. The realization would be all the more threatening because they've been there; they've seen the inside of a skull welling with brain tissue and spinal fluid that can't be put back. Most of us deal only with the shut surgery door and the camouflage of white bandages after the wounds have been cleaned and closed. We deal with secondary sources and the messengers. But doctors deal with primary sources and the full if often unacknowledged understanding of what they cannot accomplish, and what can go wrong.

The good doctors, the healers, use this knowledge to help their patients. In their attempts to protect themselves from such knowledge, the technicians don't.

13
Docs in the Manger

The good guys and the bad guys—the medical echelons of cancer treatment have both. You might encounter only the occasional bad egg, a peripheral player easily by-passed. Or you might stumble directly into the orbit of a doctor who only adds to the misery. Although usually well-intentioned, such doctors either never had, or have lost, the healing touch. Patients talk of the anger, the sense of betrayal, the heartbreak, when the doctor they had looked to for help doesn't come through. Sometimes, the patient's expectations are too high, looking for their doctors to be superhuman—tireless, infallible, and able to perform miracles. And sometimes doctors do play god, but not the sort you'd want running your universe. These are the ones who treat you as a test tube. These are the ones who have no time to answer your questions or try to reassure you. These are the ones who withdraw hope. And these are the docs in the manger who will not sanction, or even consider, other approaches, even when their own have failed.

In an ideal world, cancer patients and their doctors work together in a partnership, the sole goal to beat or at least to control the cancer. Teamwork. Makes sense. And it happens for many patients. When Woolly Setteducato had his first surgery, no one expected him to survive: the double whammy of a heart condition and cancer throughout his body left only a tiny glimmer of hope. It flickered brightly enough to get Woolly through the operation. He survived. When he thanked the surgeon for saving his life, the response was, "Not me, Woolly. *You* and me. We are a team. You wanted to live."

After his second surgery two and a half years later for what his physicians were convinced was metastatic cancer, that same surgeon greeted him with the good news. "No cancer, just scar tissue." Woolly tried to thank him again. "Don't thank me," the doctor said. "Nothing to do with me. Thank those people in the Bahamas. They did it, not me. Get back there as soon as you can."

The psychological support of this doctor was surely as important as his surgical skills.

Edwina Smith, in her seven-year-and-holding battle with germ-cell ovarian cancer, has worked with several oncologists and surgeons, consulting, discussing, and ultimately making her own decisions, but almost always with support and input from her doctors. Even when she told her team that she wanted to try an unconventional treatment—vaccine therapy—they hung in there with her. She said, "I don't want any more chemo. I've had it. I'm looking for other options. . . . And that's tricky, when you decide to step away from conventional medicine. . . . I concluded after a fair amount of digging around and reading and going on the Internet and everything that . . . I wanted to try vaccine therapy." The partnership survived even this turn of events.

One of her doctors had already told her that immune-boosting treatments would not help with germ-cell cancer because it's too aggressive, and works too fast. Edwina's response was from the heart: "Because I was chemo-exhausted, I basically said, 'I don't care if it has any promise, I'm doing something, and it ain't chemo . . . because I can't go back there right now.' And I can't believe the support I had . . . [My oncologists] said, 'I think it's a good next step; you want to try it, I'll do it with you'. . . . That was a terrific step of faith on their part. I mean you can't ask for [better] co-fighters. . . . I think there are troubles with our medical system, but it sure isn't with the people that I've encountered. . . . apart from a few jerks. I think there are MAJOR problems with the way we treat cancer but I don't think it's with the people."

Unfortunately, the experiences of Woolly and Edwina are not the norm when it comes to support for an alternative route.

The stories you most often hear are of those patients who do not have their doctors' blessing when they stray from the fold of the medical establishment, even when they are fighting late-stage malignant disease or a cancer that has shown no response to chemotherapy or radiation. The question comes up over and over in conversations with patients: Why do doctors do this? Even if they don't actively support me, couldn't they at least listen? If they have nothing to offer in their own treatment arsenal, why are they so reluctant to help, or at least not hinder, a patient who wants to search in another? In some cases, doctors consider it unethical to support "unproven" treatment; some think further experimental chemotherapy within the confines of a clinical trial is infinitely better than anything outside it; some seem to think it preferable for a patient to do nothing at all rather than try an alternative therapy; and some don't appear to think at all. Patients talk of their doctors' knee-jerk reaction to even the most timid of queries about alternatives.

Don Butterworth of St. John's, Newfoundland, recounts his experience. He was feeling miserable, thought he had the flu. He was working on the Hibernia oil project at the time, in quality control/assurance. A good place to incubate flu. When the flu wouldn't go away, he was treated for pneumonia. When the pneumonia wouldn't go away, he was sent for chest X-rays which indicated a collapsed lung. When a CT scan showed nothing, the surgeon opted for a thoracotomy: After the operation, the surgeon said, "Looks good to me. But we have one more test." In fact, the medical records show that the surgery revealed that Don was full of cancer. "The surgeon knew then, but maybe was buying time for himself," Don says. "He didn't want to give me the bad news."

After he learned that he had an untreatable cancer, mesothelioma, Don's next appointment was with the oncologist at the cancer clinic who told him that all they could do for him was to register him at the clinic so that they could give him morphine to control the pain from the surgery.

He and his wife, Robin, started to research other methods of treatment, since nothing was available in conventional treatment. Don says that when they asked the surgeon about immunotherapy, his response was, "Hey, if you are thinking about going that route, you need a psychiatrist."

This doctor, in a few sentences, has told his patient that (1) he has cancer; (2) it is untreatable; (3) he has less than a year to live; and (4) he is nuts if he tries to do anything else about it.

Most practitioners, however they deliver the message, truly believe they are protecting their patients from quackery, from financial ruin, and from further disappointment. For example, Dr. David Stewart, head of medical oncology at the Ottawa

Regional Cancer Centre, cautions about presenting experimental therapies as *the* cure. "It's important not to give people false hope because they might make inappropriate decisions" (Lau 1999, p. 16).

When a doctor refuses to condone, or at least consider, a patient's choice to pursue treatment beyond the mainstream, most patients don't care what the doctor's motivation is; they perceive it as cruel and unusual punishment. On top of battling the disease, they feel they now are at war with their own medical team, a fight that saps any energy they may have left. A doctor's refusal even to consider any other possibility not only slams the door on hope, it increases the spiraling fear and feelings of helplessness, especially in patients who have just been told there is nothing more that can be done for them.

To her conventional doctors, Annabel Brown's decision to go to the IAT Clinic was "inappropriate." She pitted her frail strength against the weight of Toronto's biggest cancer treatment hospital to get herself there. Annabel was diagnosed with malignant melanoma in 1994. "I was at Princess Margaret Hospital. They were wonderful. They were really wonderful," Annabel says about her initial treatment and support. After a major skin graft she had no more treatment until 1996, when shortness of breath alerted her to another problem. After many tests, a bronchoscopy, a pleuroscopy, and three visits for fluid drainage from the pleural cavity, she was finally diagnosed: it wasn't a metastasis from the original melanoma but a new cancer altogether—mesothelioma.

Mesothelioma is one of the rarer cancers in adulthood. It begins in either the linings that cover the lungs (the pleura) or the lining that covers the bowel and inside of the abdomen. "Most cases of mesothelioma are related to asbestos exposure" (Buckman, 1995, p. 292). Annabel had been puzzled by this. "They told me asbestos was the probable source but where I had picked up asbestos is anybody's guess." When Annabel was a small child her father worked in the shipyards of Glasgow during the war. According to Buckman, not only people who work directly with asbestos are at risk, but also their families, because of "small particles of asbestos brought home on the worker's clothing or skin." Annabel says, "Another source was our gas masks. I had a gas mask as a child during the war. But my doctors say that is too long ago. You never know. You never know."

Her surgeon at first suggested removing the pleura. "Now, this is major, major surgery. To remove the pleura, I mean, it's attached to all the ribs, the peritoneum, the pericardium around the heart. And the lung would go too." But when they discovered cancer in her left lung as well as on the right side, surgery was out of the question. And generally, mesotheliomas do not respond to chemotherapy or radiation.

Annabel says, "They finally said, 'I'm sorry we can't do anything for you. When you start having symptoms . . . then we can perhaps treat you.'

"So, I went home. It took me a few days to figure out what they had really said." Annabel laughs. "It didn't register too quickly. 'Go home and die.' I thought, I don't like this. I don't want to sit around and wait until I start having symptoms. I asked them what the symptoms were. One doctor said, 'We won't tell you, because then you'll start having them.'"

Once a mesothelioma diagnosis is made, "Death commonly ensues within one year" (Clement, 1988). Annabel had so little time. The statistical probabilities gave her a few months at best, months she did not want to spend waiting passively for death. She wanted to look at all possibilities, to see if she could defy those probabilities. Other people had.

She read about the IAT Clinic and its apparent success with mesothelioma patients. A study of eleven mesothelioma patients on immuno-augmentative therapy between May 1980 and February 1987 found that the therapy "affect[s] survival favorably . . . the mean survival of these patients ranged from 7–80 months with mean and median survivals of 35 months and 30 months respectively." The study, published in 1988 and updated in 1998, was written by Dr. John Clement and based on direct clinical experience. All these patients had been originally diagnosed at hospitals or diagnostic centers other than the IAT Clinic. This is important to note, since a common criticism of claims of treatment success by alternative methods is that the patients in question never had cancer in the first place. In 1999, three of these patients are still alive. Although "[t]here are no published series in which matched groups of patients have been subjected to a variety of treatments," Clement quotes the results of several other small studies of mesothelioma patients treated with conventional therapies that indicate much lower survival rates. For example, a study of six patients treated at the Sidney Farber Cancer Institute and the Peter Bent Brigham Hospital in the United States revealed a median survival of fifteen months from diagnosis to death (Antman et al. 1980).

When Annabel raised the idea of going to IAT, her doctor at Princess Margaret "grew quite angry, quite agitated, said that he would absolutely not support my going there. Even though they couldn't do anything for me, they didn't want me to go anywhere else, especially this alternative clinic."

With gentle conviction, Annabel stuck to her decision.

When patients opt for an alternative treatment, sometimes they need more than their doctor's blessing. In the new field of cancer vaccines, the patient's tumor material is necessary to build that vaccine. Sometimes this is even harder to come by than a doctor's reluctant approval to go that route.

In Ottawa, Sue McPherson was told by her doctors that there was nothing more they could do for her—after surgeries, radiation treatments, and chemotherapy, her various cancers had won (leukemia, radiation-induced thyroid cancer, and metastatic breast cancer, a linear invasion of cellular proliferation that eventually took over her body and defeated her spirit). They gave her two months to live. Sue wanted more than two months, but the prognosis seemed to become a self-fulfilling prophecy for her. Not so for her family and friends. In the face of her waning strength, Sue gave two friends medical power of attorney to help her sort out what to do next. She was exhausted by her disease, by her treatment, and by an assortment of doctors who, to her, appeared uncomprehending and unsympathetic. We can't do anything more for you. Goodbye.

One of her friends heard about Immunocomp, an experimental anticancer vaccine that was available in Ottawa through Bill O'Neill's Canadian Cancer Research Group. Health Canada allowed its entry from the United States under the Therapeutic Products Program (TPP). To make up the vaccine, the laboratory in Stockbridge, Georgia, needed tumor material from Sue. This meant a biopsy. There began a four-month struggle with the hospital and doctors in Ottawa—two months more than Sue was supposed to have—to get the biopsy done. The delays at first seemed of the usual bureaucratic variety— no operating rooms available, waiting lists for "elective" surgery, and so on. But then surgeons began to toss the case back and forth: "I can't do a rib surgery and that's where the biopsy should come from. I can only do hips," was what she and her friends heard at one appointment. New tests and scans suddenly were required. What was going on here?

Sue's friends went into high gear, insisted on meetings with all the surgeons involved, and finally got action. The biopsy was performed—a two-hour operation to remove a part of Sue's rib. The surgeon came out into the hospital concourse where Sue's family and friends waited. In his hand, he held a bloody portion of bone, wrapped in a cloth. "Come with me to the pathology lab," he said to the horrified friend. "You want some of this." She went with him while he sawed the rib in two pieces, handing her one, which she placed in a thermos she had brought with her. It is difficult to believe that if that tumor material had been destined for Johns Hopkins or the Princess Margaret Hospital it would have been delivered in such an off-hand—and unsterile—fashion.

When Carolyn Widger from Wilton, Connecticut, was diagnosed with ovarian cancer, stage 4, in August 1996, she had massive surgery: "The surgeon was wonderful; he saved my life," she says.

Next step: stem-cell transplant. "I didn't know much about this, I didn't know it would completely destroy my immune system." She went back to the hospital for her second bout of chemotherapy . . . and walked out. "This is all wrong for my body. There has to be an alternative," she thought.

When she arrived at the IAT Clinic her blood cell count was so dangerously low that the clinic sent her back to the States for a bone-marrow biopsy to see what was going on. "My oncologist in Connecticut has been a star about all this, very supportive, but not real happy about me coming to the Bahamas," she says. But he was there for her, supported her decision. To save her the trip all the way back to Connecticut, he recommended a doctor in Florida to whom she could go for the biopsy. When the Florida doctor heard she was at the IAT Clinic he refused to take her on as a patient. He was "very angry" that she was returning to the Bahamas, would not write a prescription for Neupogen shots for her, would not send biopsy results to IAT, or even give them to her. He would, however, send them to her oncologist in Connecticut.

The Florida doctor told her, "They don't cure anyone at IAT."

Carolyn said, "But I've met people who have been coming back to the clinic for years after they had been told they had only months to live by their own doctors."

His response was, "Then they probably didn't have cancer in the first place."

But these patients have all been diagnosed in their home towns, in their own treating hospitals, well within the conventional bulwarks.

Braxton Colley's oncologist said the same thing, but neither he nor Carolyn's doctor could explain the inordinate number of patients "misdiagnosed" in their own hospitals, all of whom seemed to have ended up at IAT. When Colley's oncologist saw the tracking tests after his first IAT treatments which indicated that the cancer had been stabilized, he said that Braxton probably had never had mesothelioma in the first place. But how could that be? Colley's medical records from the hospital that diagnosed him read as follows: "right thoracotomy, a wedge biopsy of the lower lobe and pleura was obtained which showed malignant mesothelioma." And it was mesothelioma that this same oncologist was trying to eradicate with chemotherapy. If he didn't have this cancer, then just what was this oncologist treating him for?

Another interpretation would be that he and these other doctors were trying to prevent harm, by discouraging a patient from pursuing an "unproven" treatment. But what price "proven"? Braxton Colley and so many other cancer patients see the price as their own lives, far too high to pay even for the common good. Were Carolyn and Braxton, Steve and Marcia, Lena and Dave and all the other IAT patients wrong to choose immuno-augmentative therapy, which has no side effects (and, according to most conventional practitioners, no other effects either) over chemotherapy, with its horrific side effects (which, according to other critics, are also its *only* effects)? Their physicians back home thought so. Better to go with the minuscule odds of experimental and debilitating therapy *within* the scientific parameters, than *any* therapy outside them.

As Gerald Lampe asked at the Molinari congressional hearing on the IAT Clinic: "[b]y the Oath of Hippocrates, physicians are commanded to 'do no harm' to their patients by commission or omission. This command has been ignored and harm has been done to thousands by omitting truth and open selection of choices. . . . Given the poor performance and usually difficult side effects of chemotherapy, it is difficult to understand why it is yet promoted as the treatment of choice and promise to the dying patient." (Wright 1985, p. 85).

Why then *is* it promoted? Why do doctors think that you, as patient, should stick with the "proven" therapies, whatever the odds? You will hear at least three answers to those questions. It helps to stamp out quackery; it provides the patients and families with at least the illusion that something is being done; and there is a remote, statistical possibility that it might work.

"[F]or some forms of cancer, chemotherapy results in palliation for brief duration in 5–10 percent of the cases. . . . Nevertheless, chemotherapy serves an extremely valuable role in keeping patients oriented toward proper medical therapy, and prevents the feeling of being abandoned by the physician in patients with late and hopeless cancers. Judicious employment and screening of potentially useful drugs may also prevent the spread of quackery. . . . Properly based chemotherapy can serve a useful purpose in preventing improper orientation of the patient" (Richards 1972, p. 215, quoted in Moss 1995, p. 164).

Dr. Groopman, Recanati professor of immunology at Harvard Medical School and chief of experimental medicine at Beth Israel Deaconess Medical Center, agrees that chemotherapy is often administered for the wrong reasons; he does not condone the practice. "To treat for the sake of treating, when there is no hope of the toxic drugs having a significant effect on the disease, is an all-too-common practice among physicians. It is rationalized as giving the patient and his loved ones comfort from the appearance of *something* being done, but in truth it only increases suffering. I would not condone such a course" (1997, p. 118).

Finally, for those oncologists who encourage their patients to take chemotherapy because it might extend their lives for a few months—advice based on a tiny statistical possibility—this might prop up a system, but certainly takes its toll on the individual.

In many cases (though not all), these doctors are acting out of a misplaced humanity. Their experience, their education, their instincts all say that the cancer is way ahead of the treatment and that death is imminent. The person in their care is going to die, and they must be the conveyers of this stark message. If they are truthful and deliver the message, they are perceived not as realists but as heartless, uncaring monsters. They cannot face tolling the death knell. It is not sadism or rule books but their own humanity and personal squeamishness that lead them into the deception of ordering more treatment. It is an irony that doing so often leads to more, not less, suffering for the very person they are trying to help. They feel that doing something—anything—as long as it is within the confines of conventional treatment, is better than doing nothing. So they order up more chemo, higher doses of radiation. These are the tools they have been taught are the only tools. The tunnel vision induced by the rigid parameters of their medical training traps them and their patients in the killing fields of convention.

For the doctor in Florida to refuse Carolyn Widger as a patient because she had ventured beyond the conventional boundaries is restricting access to medical treatment—a flagrant abuse of patients' rights.

For Sue McPherson's surgeon to so casually wave about a piece of cancerous rib in the hospital waiting room in front of her family was an act of monumental disrespect, apparently because the owner of that rib had dared to venture into the alternative treatment world.

For Braxton Colley's oncologist to encourage him to take an experimental chemotherapy in the full knowledge that it was not going to touch the mesothelioma, particularly if he truly believed that Colley had been misdiagnosed, comes close to malpractice.

An elderly man lies dying of lung cancer in a Vancouver hospital. He has been on chemotherapy for two years. He has also had radiation. Both appear to have helped, in that they have at least extended his life. His family says, "They fried his brain. But it was successful because the cancer didn't go there." But now, he's had enough. He's tired; he's nauseated from the chemo, burned by the radiation. He wants the treatment discontinued. He wants to be left in peace.

His family tell the doctor, "No more chemo." But the doctor insists. Why? Perhaps because of his medical training, but that is no excuse. For at least a decade, there have been strong voices crying out against exactly what this doctor was doing. As

Albert Braverman noted in *The Lancet*: "Chemotherapy should be prescribed only when there is a reasonable prospect either of cure or of benefit in quantity and quality of life. [O]ncology trainees should be taught that chemotherapy is not part of the management of every cancer patient" (1991, p. 901).

The above story illustrates so many of the issues cancer patients face, issues that have little to do with their actual disease and much to do with the wrongs that exist in cancer treatment today.

First, of course, is the brutality of the treatment itself: to give up on life not because of the disease but because of the suffering caused by its treatment is a sorry comment on the state of cancer therapy. Despite amazing new anti-nausea drugs and improved pain-control methods, the fact remains that chemotherapy is no picnic. The drugs are toxic, designed to destroy cancer cells. Unfortunately, they are unselective in their onslaught, damaging so much else in the body.

Then there is the blatant abuse of patients' rights: the patient has the right to say, "Stop the treatment." But this doctor ignored his wishes. Did this doctor really believe he could "cure" his patient at this late stage? Or extend his life a little longer? At what cost? For the patient, it was no longer a life worth living. Or did the doctor see this as an opportunity to test a different drug, perhaps still in the experimental stages? With a terminal patient, this is sometimes authorized, but only with the knowledge of the patient and his family.

This doctor might have been afraid of a lawsuit, understandable in these increasingly litigious times. Perhaps he insisted on administering more chemo through fear of being charged with negligence or, indeed, even manslaughter for not "treating" the patient to the very end.

Such a motive doesn't necessarily get you home free, though. Doctors must be increasingly frustrated by the "tails you lose, heads you lose" world they find themselves in. A public inquiry was held in February 1999 in Montreal into the death of Herman Krausz, a seventy-six-year-old patient at the Jewish General Hospital who died fifteen hours after doctors took him off the respirator. Krausz's family and hospital officials have conflicting versions of why the decision was made. The doctors said it was because they had determined that his condition was irreversible. The family said that, though they knew Mr. Krausz was going to die, the doctors acted against his and the family's wishes, and that they had no right to turn off the respirator to hasten his death.

It appears as if the players in both these deathbed dramas fell headlong into what is euphemistically called "the communications gap," a bland phrase for the hellish situation the patient finds himself in at the end of his life. The doctors in Vancouver did not take the time to explain the treatment. Or if they did, they did not ensure that the family and patient understood what they were saying. The man's family described his radiation treatments as "frying the brain" to prevent it from "catching" cancer. Even the most committed of radiologists would balk at administering such treatment. Perhaps the radiation was given because of metastasis to the brain; perhaps the radiation was aimed at another part of the head or neck. But whatever the reason, the patient and his family deserved to know what was happening to him, and why.

In Mr. Krausz's situation, it also seems the doctors weren't listening. They either ignored his wishes, or perhaps hadn't heard him over the swoosh and hum of technology—and in the silence after they pulled the plug, it was too late.

No wonder medical students are shying away from choosing cancer treatment as their area of speciality. The outcomes are too uncertain. No glory, little glamor, and impossible decisions. Damned if you do, damned if you don't. Doctors are blamed for continuing to treat a patient in the last stages of cancer; they are also blamed if they say, "That's it, there is nothing more we can do for you." Terrible to have to deliver such a message, but worse to have to receive it. And yet the fear and grief at being told it is the end of the line may be compounded by what often is a brutal conveyance of that message, along with the slamming of the door on any other possible route.

Don Butterworth describes how his doctor told him that he had untreatable, terminal cancer: "It was the shortest doctor's appointment I've ever had. I came in, sat down. The surgeon looked down at the floor and said, 'I hate this part of my job. I'm sorry, there is nothing we can do for you. You have mesothelioma. Good luck.'

"I said, 'Wait, let's get our cards out on the table here. How much time do I have?'

"The surgeon replied, 'I've never seen a meso patient live longer than a year after diagnosis. That's it. Goodbye.' And he walked out of the room."

He later suggested that Don might be losing his marbles for even considering going to an immunology clinic.

Don and Sue and Annabel chose to continue to fight against their disease, however, even after their doctors said there was no point. To "keep patients oriented toward proper medical therapy" and "to prevent the spread of quackery" are two sides of the same coin: both are sacrificing individual needs to a system. To deny these patients support in finding another therapy that might, just might, help them, and certainly would not harm them, in order to keep them oriented toward proper medical therapy makes no sense. "Proper medical therapy" had already failed them.

When Faye Pennington arrived at the IAT Clinic she was fleeing from her doctor's death sentence: "At this point the only thing that I know is that we are just going to make you as comfortable as we can for the time you have left." Between 1980 and 1982, she had had twenty radiation treatments and eleven months of chemo for lymphoma, but her cancer just continued to spread. She had almost given up hope. Certainly her doctor had. Dr. Burton told her that the IAT treatment would help her (not "cure" her, but help her body gain control of her cancer). "When he told me that, it gave me something to live for. . . . When the Lord showed me this place and I came down here, it gave me power to overcome what I had been told. I got back my joy." For "joy" read "hope." That was seventeen years ago.

When Bill O'Neill talks about patients who turn to alternative therapies, he says, "These patients are flocking to a number of things and the first thing is hope. The clinical oncologists will call it false hope. Hope cannot be qualified. Hope is simply something better for tomorrow. Anyone who interferes with that, anyone who tampers with it, is, I believe, morally and ethically responsible for injuring the patient."

The simplistic acceptance that all conventional doctors are the Bad Guys, all alternative practitioners are the Good Guys, or vice versa, does everyone a disservice. It doesn't work like that. There is a mix, a blurring across the lines. On *60 Minutes* a man with a brain tumor summed it up: "The mistake is that people think all doctors are the same. That is wrong. There are good doctors and there are bad doctors, just as in any other profession. Yet medicine is the only profession where we expect all practitioners to be the same."

We accept that there are good lawyers, there are bad lawyers; there are dishonest lawyers, there are lazy lawyers. We shop around for a good architect, get referrals, look at their work. With doctors we rarely shop around; we accept unquestioningly their edicts. We've been hiring or firing lawyers for centuries; but it's only recently we have begun to talk about hiring or firing a doctor.

Most doctors aren't villains—they don't set out to make people suffer needlessly. But sometimes their humanity is overwhelmed by other considerations. In such cases, and if you are physically able, it is time for you to fire your doctor and find another who resists technology in the consultation room, who is open to possibilities outside his or her ken, who sees you as a person, rather than a disease, who knows how to preserve hope, and who understands healing. It is a tall order.

14

Patient Responsibility: Gift or Burden?

Hand in hand with freedom of choice goes patient responsibility, perhaps even a thornier issue, not so much for medical authorities as for the patients themselves. Nowadays, people facing a cancer diagnosis are less likely to accept without demur the doctor's decision on their treatment. They question, they research, they talk to other patients, they go for second or even third medical opinions. They take responsibility for their own health care. For some, this route works. For others, it is a Pandora's box, releasing an avalanche of information which becomes a burden rather than an empowerment. They would rather keep the lid firmly shut on the plethora of choices and just do what the doctor says. Still others make their choice based not on information, not on doctors' orders or advice, but on instinct, a gut reaction to the options available.

After surgery and eight months of chemotherapy, recommended by my doctors, and certainly not questioned by me, I had to confront the patient responsibility issue. This was a new world. *I*, not my doctors, had to decide whether to go the whole hog and have radiation too. The Tumor Board of three doctors met, discussed my case, and did not reach consensus. They had no clear recommendation so it was up to me. I was given all the information: radiation would prevent recurrence to the original tumor site; it would not have an impact on possible recurrence anywhere else. It was not an invasive treatment and it would have few side effects. If I had it now, I could never have radiation treatment again on the same part of my body, since I would be getting the maximum RADs the human body can tolerate. Uh-huh. Uh-huh. I heard the words, but they were meaningless, snared in a brain made stagnant by chemo and confusion. I wanted the doctors to agree with each other, to tell me with assurance what I should do, and I wanted them to be right. It didn't work that way.

Unable to analyze, to make connections, to use information upon which to decide, I did the next best thing. I based my decision on a dream. Was it the right decision? Who knows? It was right for me, at the time. There is no route that is categorically right or wrong; the right one is the one you choose. Often, the toughest part is being resolute in your choice, hanging on to the courage of your original commitment, and if things don't go well, resisting the temptation to second-guess your choice.

This decade has its health care buzzwords. The most popular is "prevention"—it's up to you to stay healthy—followed closely by "patient responsibility" and "taking control." In cancer treatment, they can provide a sense of strength and direction, or they can lead to confusion, frustration, and guilt.

The experiences of two cancer patients illustrate the power and pitfalls in this relatively recent trend toward patient participation.

Edwina's story is an example of how making decisions in a proactive partnership with the medical team can help achieve that delicate balance amid contradictions that living with cancer requires. Her story is a kind of intelligent woman's guide to the cancer treatment galaxy. Rachel's experience illustrates, first, the conundrum of cancer treatment when research and practice get out of sync, forcing the patient to base a major decision on the ephemeral "proof" of probabilities and statistics that contradict each other. And second, her experience captures the frustration of being forced into the driver's seat, not because she wanted to manage her own health care but because no one else was.

When Edwina Smith learned from her own research that there was a 95 percent statistical probability that she could be cured of her disease—germ-cell cancer of the ovaries—it was easy to go with the doctors' decision for her to have surgery and chemotherapy. When the cancer came back, the subsequent decisions became more difficult, and they became hers.

Her journey, so far, spans seven years and as many different treatments, remissions, and recurrences, numerous doctors, a support group, and family members unwavering in their support and commitment to her. She travels a difficult path, quietly taking responsibility for her life, enlisting help from all sides with grace and humor and dignity. "In all these years," she says, "I have had only three bad experiences with the medical profession. I have been so lucky in my caregivers." Not just lucky: Edwina's gift is that she can turn the negative experiences into positive ones, not in a Pollyanna sort of way, but by flipping them around and making them work in her favor.

In the summer of 1992, Edwina felt so unwell her GP sent her for an ultrasound. It revealed an abdominal mass the size of a grapefruit. She was booked for surgery three weeks later. (The speed with which the operation was scheduled did not indicate an emergency—keep in mind that this was in the days before our health system slipped into crisis mode. Her gynecologist was reassuring; it's 99 percent certain to be a benign cyst on the ovary, he told her. Go home, rest, don't worry. What she did was go home and watch her stomach grow. She called her gynecologist: "Listen, I know that we've got surgery scheduled for December 16 or something, but I just want you to know while you're sticking to this schedule, this thing is growing."

"Impossible," he said.

"It took a lot of courage to make that phone call," Edwina says, "because you grow up with, you know, 'Doctor knows everything.' Well, I had the surgery, and to his credit, the first thing he said was, 'I owe you a very sincere apology. You were in fact right. It is growing, because you have a very aggressive, very malignant cancer.' That was my very first lesson: you're dealing with people working within a frame of reference of their own training . . . their decision making is guided by probability rather than certainty."

The probability was that the growth was a benign cyst; the certainty was that it was growing like a mushroom, which benign cysts normally don't do. It was the probability that blinkered the doctor, making him reject Edwina's observation of her own body. The mass was growing very fast and she knew it. The cancer she has is one of the fastest-growing there is.

"But I have great admiration for this doctor," Edwina says. "It was a huge admission for him to say, 'I'm sorry.' He was very kind to me, came to visit every day."

At about this time she learned another lesson in coping. It came with the resident who visited her before her surgery. "This sweet young thing asks me to sign this consent form; now I'm not even thirty-five yet and I'm looking at this *teenager*; the issue for me, because I'm this eternal optimist, wasn't that I was going to be fatally ill from the cancer but it was the possibility of having to have a full hysterectomy. . . . When this young resident asked me to sign a consent that basically gave them the right to clean out all of my reproductive organs depending on what they would find, I asked him, 'Are you doing the surgery?'"

"Oh, no, no, I don't do the surgery."

And I said, "Well, I'm not signing anything until I talk to the man who's actually making the decision at the table." That was another hard thing to do.

This was not about an insensitive or stupid resident, Edwina says, but, "It's the system. It's set up for efficiency; it's about getting the paperwork done. The surgeon—the man making the decision at the table—did come in and talk to me; it had been his intention all along. It was just that the bureaucracy got there first."

After surgery, with the help of friends and family, she researched and read everything she could, then went to her medical appointments with a list of questions and one or two of her brothers. "I needed to understand." And she needed to be sure she heard the answers right. Her brothers were her ears, her sounding boards; they sieved everything out but the nuggets of facts and options she needed to make her next choice.

With her 95 percent cure prognosis, Edwina did not at first question the medical route planned for her: "[M]y coping then and the kind of decisions and the kind of involvement that I had was to find out as much as I could about the cancer, to get some reassurance from the reading, and then to learn how to manage the treatment. The crucial decision making in terms of what drugs, what surgery, I left entirely to my oncologist. I was very comfortable with that . . . at the time."

She points out ruefully that such a rare cancer tends to fascinate doctors; they are intrigued and willing to give it a lot of attention. But that is not the only reason for their support; much of the success of this partnership lies in Edwina's approach. She makes the partnership work for her by being "someone who could speak objectively . . . not using all the medical language but with the attitude of the clinician, which is objective . . . that was my approach by nature, it wasn't something I adopted deliberately. . . . I would say that in the first nine months of treatment and the follow-up appointments, I was sort of a classic well-informed person. I wanted the physician to make the decisions, but I wanted to be extremely well-informed, to understand and participate in my own care at home. And I was never really that afraid because my chances were so good for a cure. My biggest concern, actually, was coping with everyone else's fear."

When she finished treatment that first time, she was basically told, "Go off and live your life, you're cured. Which I did. Had a great time. But I made major life changes. . . . I quit my job and I got a house and I went on trips and off I went."

But Edwina was not cured by surgery and chemotherapy. When her cancer came back less than two years later, her partnership with her doctors took on a different and more permanent hue. Again, Edwina set the tone: "If I went in there organized, able to talk calmly, able to shelve my emotional struggle and leave it behind, then the relationships worked well and I felt that as much partnership as I asked for I received."

This time, though, her doctors were more guarded in their prognosis: "My oncologist was very kind, but made it very clear that once you've relapsed, 'cure' is not a word you're going to hear. To be honest, though, I don't remember accepting that. I thought, maybe, maybe—for someone else. . . ."

So Edwina was willing to take more chemotherapy. And more. And more.

After seven or eight cycles of tougher and tougher chemotherapy, after a full hysterectomy, after a bone-marrow transplant, like the damn cat, the cancer still came back.

Until her second relapse, Edwina says, she would go to her doctors and say, "OK, now what are you going to do to get me through this?" But the recurrences changed that: she didn't want to be ruled anymore, either by her doctors or her disease. She recognized that her doctors had the education, certainly, "but frankly they don't have any decisions that they can make that are any more important than mine."

> I was learning by then that physicians are only people,
> [I was] learning that cancer may be a death sentence,
> but that you can live for a long time with cancer, that
> you can accommodate it, that you can even live joyfully
> with it, and that you can survive the treatments . . .
> [I was learning] that the more informed, assertive,
> thoughtful you are about your own care, the more
> involvement you have, the more opportunity you have
> to coexist with cancer more successfully. . . . You
> develop this bifocal thing where on the one hand
> you're very aware of the fact that you will probably
> die from cancer and in probably a pretty uncomfort-
> able way. That's a fact in your life. It's underneath
> everything that you do. At the same time, and no less
> convinced, you know that you can beat it. So you
> accept this contradiction. It's not vacillation. They're
> two completely opposite convictions that you live
> with every day. And that feeds into all of your decision
> making. It was important for me to recognize that
> dichotomy because it became the way I assessed my
> choices . . . if in fact the cancer's going to kill me, do
> I want to spend the last three months of my life sick
> as a dog and unable to be me? . . . I look at a treatment
> and say this may be the one that'll kick me into a cure

and if it doesn't, am I willing to pay the price? And they all have big price tags, very high price tags. Because the price tag isn't physical suffering. It's that the physical suffering takes you out of your life. It completely undermines who you are, your person-hood, your relationships. When you're nauseated and can barely stand up because your body is so weak, and you're so nauseated you can hardly hold a con-versation, who are you? And that was always, that was always the horror of it. The horror of the decid-ing if the chemo does not work, if the next treatment doesn't work, do I really want to spend my last six months in that condition.

One of the toughest decisions was whether to have the bone-marrow transplant. "[W]hat I was struggling with and didn't know it, was I had no criteria." But during the two ago-nizing weeks she had to make the decision (it is a risky pro-cedure at the best of times and for Edwina doubly so because she had been weakened by so much chemotherapy), she found that she was developing a framework she still uses today. "It isn't simply an either/or; it's a framework that relies on rela-tionships with my physicians, my family, it's not a formula."

Her doctors helped her with the process of decision mak-ing, rather than advising her on the decisions themselves. They spent hours with her, on the phone, at meetings held at her request. "They had the wisdom from their own experience with other patients to know what I was going through and they used that wisdom for my benefit." "Think about your body as a bank account," one told her. "And think about how much you want to draw on that bank account, because every treatment takes something away from you." That was a turning point for her.

I guess maybe there are four things that go into the mix. The first one is what is the likelihood of my getting a period of health after this treatment that would make it worthwhile? The guideline I use is if I invest a month of illness, I want a month of health. The second one is how much is this treatment going to take out of my physical bank account that means I can't pursue another alternative if it doesn't work? ...

The third one is, what is it going to be like to live through the treatment? What burden is it going to place on me and the people around me, and am I willing to pay that price? You know, do I want to be sick . . . to that extent? And the fourth one to me is really so fundamental: How hopeful do I feel? What is my gut telling me? Does this make me feel, you know, this could actually work. Life's going to happen for me. I could walk away from this. Or do I feel like, you know, it might only give me a couple of months. . . . It's very instinctive.

And of the four ingredients in the decision-making mix, which is the most important?

"Hopefulness, without question. But I don't arrive there unless I go through the other three. I'm one of those people who sounds indecisive—'Maybe I should . . . and what if I did? . . . and if I don't?' But that's a process and at the end of it, when I've decided, I never look back . . . And every other decision after the [bone-marrow transplant] was easier because of the tools I had developed."

After the first recurrence of her cancer, Edwina did something she had resisted before. Because she isn't much of a joiner, because she's a private person who likes doing things on her own, she avoided the whole idea of support groups as hokey. Too touchy-feely. Didn't want to spend time with people who were probably just going to die. To appease a friend who had extracted a promise from her to go at least once, she went to one meeting and was hooked. It turned out to be one of the best decisions she could have made.

> If you ask me what are the two things that have helped me manage, I would say it's been the support of family and friends and the support group, because it is the only place I can get certain kinds of hope, and it's the only place I can get certain kinds of information that give hope.

The combination of the group, her family, and her friends create a safety net for her.

> [F]amily and friends are who give me joy, and that to me is what surviving and thriving is all about, why you can make those tough decisions with a fair amount of serenity. It doesn't mean it's easy, but those are the things that help you determine the criteria with which you're going to make decisions. . . . They grow within you, they become part of who you are. You know you will do this, but not do that. You will try this, but not try that. You will push the envelope only in certain directions on certain conditions. And as treatment after treatment fails, those things become more and more important, because [the cancer] no longer is an enemy that's over there somewhere that you're fighting. It has become something that's ruling your entire life.

Edwina takes responsibility for her own decisions, "I think everybody's response is very individual and over time and with experience, you start to learn your own patterns. I think it's very important to learn your own coping mechanisms and what gives you ease and what doesn't, what makes a decision easier to make or what gives you peace of mind. . . . In terms of making decisions, the single most important thing I have done is work in partnership." She has also assumed responsibility for taking advantage of all the resources she can find in her fight to keep cancer from controlling her life, including joining a support group: "[A]s you face the issues more and more and become more comfortable with them, it's harder and harder to talk to people who haven't been through it." What they say in comfort and support can't capture the contradictions. People who have or have had cancer know how multi-dimensional the experience is and how deep it runs.

She has drawn together what she needs, even managing to find gold in the dross of some of her medical encounters including the one with the specialist who chewed her out for having the temerity to bring a list of questions with her about a possible bone-marrow transplant. She didn't back down in the face of his anger, although it took courage: "The fact is that these doctors have your life in their hands and it is very hard to stand up and say, 'I'm going to make you really pissed off at me.' . . . Anyway, I was proud of myself. I said, 'You know, I'm not apologizing for giving you a list of questions. This is the only way I know how to cope and understand.' To his credit, he then spent two hours with us and answered every question in fine detail. And it was, notwithstanding a horrific start, one of the most thorough consultations I've ever had."

Edwina has developed the strength of mind not to second-guess. "I've . . . had doctors say, 'You know, you shouldn't really have done that [treatment],' and I say I don't care. It was right for me then." This is a gift, as she says herself. And a rare one.

Edwina's battle continues. She has the fortitude to continue to fight, she says, because "I have not walked alone."

Two of her brothers, in particular, not only help her with decisions, they also "take care of all the clutter."

"We're a well-oiled machine now," she says ruefully. "They are my problem-solvers. They say, 'We'll manage the house, you come and live with us, we'll take care of the car, you don't have to worry about work.' When you don't have to deal with all those practical problems, you can listen to your heart. You can hear it over the worrisome noise of ordinary living. They do this for me."

And along with her doctors, her mother, other family and friends, they help her contain the emotional terror: "I guess what was running at a high-pitched scream in the early years now is a dull roar. And it doesn't shut me down anymore. But as things come up, I just have to work with them."

For many, the concept of "taking control" is frightening, a two-edged sword. Empowerment is liberating but it comes draped in responsibility, and can have a dark flip side—guilt. What happens if the way you choose doesn't work? Then how do you keep from blaming yourself? What if you choose a treatment not recommended or condoned by your doctors? Then you must contend not only with the responsibility of your own decision, but with the condemnation of your medical advisers. And what happens if you live the wrong lifestyle?

In the relentless current of the prevention and patient-responsibility movement, the opportunities for guilt are legion. Lifestyle plays a big part, and buried in lifestyle is the sharp grit of risk factors. Generally, their avoidance takes the population in a positive direction, encouraging individuals to prevent bad health through activities and choices which they themselves control. The two biggest are in the area of nutrition and exercise, with any amount of proof that both go a long way to improving health and longevity.

But the loony side to all of this is that if you accept all the dictates of the last decade of popular literature on nutrition, for instance, aside from the fact that you would be very confused by the endless debates on the goodness/badness of dairy products, red meat, wine, fat, sugar, etcetera, you might also arrive at the logical conclusion that if you followed the rules, you would live forever. And if you didn't, you would very likely develop cancer or have a heart attack or fall prey to some debilitating disease, and IT WOULD BE ALL YOUR OWN FAULT.

Well, forget that. Bad enough to have a life-threatening illness and the horrible treatments that come with it without having to feel guilty about it as well.

Risk factors for cancer are arrived at through research and observation; they are the drumbeats of the anticancer dance to which we shuffle and step. The trouble is, they keep changing. And they will keep on changing until we know what causes cancer and until we know what cures cancer. In the absence of that knowledge, it sometimes seems that cancer is becoming a behavioral disease; if we don't dance the dance, if we don't live our lives according to the edicts of risk management, then it seems we've brought the disease upon ourselves. But is this not just an attempt to propitiate the gods of a disease that we can't control, do not fully understand? Take breast cancer, for example. You hear any number of risk factors bandied about. These are the most commonly cited ones (not in any particular order):

1. Age.
2. Genetic predisposition: a history of breast cancer in the family.

3. Early menstruation and/or late menopause. (One researcher has advised giving drugs to twelve-year-old girls to delay menstruation, with the goal of reducing their risk of developing breast cancer later in life. This must be the medical equivalent of introducing one pest into the garden to eliminate another: and the only thing that gets eliminated is the garden.)
4. Long-term use of oral contraceptives.
5. Having an abortion.
6. Alcohol consumption.
7. A high-fat, low-fiber diet (five to ten servings of fruit and vegetables a day reduce the risk of cancer by 25 percent, concludes a meta-analysis of 4,500 studies in the United States).
8. Lack of exercise (according to the director of Avon Women's Running Program, you reduce your risk of breast cancer by 47 percent if you run or walk for half an hour three times a week).
9. Environmental toxins (to which you increase your exposure when you eat five to ten servings of fruits and vegetables a day!).
10. Exposure to radiation (including radiation therapy).
11. Having already had cancer.
12. Stress (not in itself a direct cause, but how the body deals with it).
13. In high-risk women, *not* taking tamoxifen. No, wait, not tamoxifen anymore, raloxifene.

Almost half of these risk factors are behavioral, carrying with them the usual slick of guilt. You can't do too much about your genetic make-up, but you certainly can exercise more, eat better, and go off the Pill. The reality is, though, the biggest risk factor of all is being a woman. Seventy-five percent of women with breast cancer have had no exposure to any other "risk factor." Except one—guilt, which certainly belongs up there in the top ten.

Look what has happened down through the history of medicine—all the leaping and writhing at the feet of a disease that took on mythical proportions until its cause and cure were nailed. Tuberculosis lost its artistic associations and romantic trappings with the advent of penicillin; gout was no longer considered a self-induced punishment for high living when it was deconstructed into a form of arthritis, the cause of which was not booze and at least eight wives.

Some risk factors are not to be denied: the genetic factor—women with the breast cancer gene have an 85 percent risk of developing the disease. However, only 8 to 10 percent of women with breast cancer are among this group. Another obvious risk is smoking and its connection with lung cancer. In this case, the risk factor is a behavioral one, controlled to a certain extent by the individual. What until recently has been carefully characterized as a theory that environmental toxins cause cancer is finally being accepted as fact. Studies are proving direct links, for instance, between the increasing incidence of breast cancer and PCBs and other organochlorines which last in the environment for decades without breaking down. Finally, the connections are being acknowledged even in the mainstream, in the face of denials by Big Industry, almost forty years after Rachel Carson warned the world about the coming of the "silent spring." But other risk factors are less credible, often nutty, and always harmful in their power to create guilt.

So you put aside the guilt, and you make choices and you don't look back. It's still not easy. As "health consumers" we are urged to make "informed" decisions, based not on instinct but on research, a truly daunting task with the glut of information now available. In public health, for example, Margaret

Somerville, the director of the Centre for Medicine, Ethics and Law at McGill University, says that the Internet is fundamentally changing how the public responds. "When you didn't have this communication, you had a black and white system," she says. "You had a very small group of people, the decision makers, who would say to the public in a paternalistic way, 'Look, we will look after you, we know best, don't you worry your little heads about it, you wouldn't understand it anyway.' That's what we call blind trust. What's happened now with our information explosion is that blind trust isn't possible anymore. People know too much" (*Ottawa Citizen*, April 29, 1996).

After being assured that our tainted-blood system was safe, that disintegrating breast implants are not a health hazard, that viruses cannot jump species (despite one theory that AIDS was unleashed on humankind through the consumption of monkeys' brains), or that "mad cow disease" is just a catchy term dreamed up by the media, we "health consumers" are flat out skeptical about any assurances coming from on high. As a society, we no longer accept the party line. As individuals faced with a cancer diagnosis we are likewise less accepting of a doctor's paternalistic advice to leave our treatment decisions to the experts. We explore and read and ask questions, but instead of coming up with a definitive answer we often come up with a fistful of contradictions. The medical certainties about cancer treatments are, in so many cases, not certainties at all, but beliefs espoused by different camps.

Tamoxifen: should it be taken by healthy women who are at high risk for developing breast cancer? North American trials say yes; European trials say no. In an interview on CBC's *The Magazine*, Hanna Gartner asked Dr. Bernard Fisher, one of the directors of the North American tamoxifen cancer-prevention trials, if women could be getting uterine cancer from taking tamoxifen to guard against breast cancer. His answer was singularly unhelpful for a woman trying to decide whether to take it: "Will the ceiling in this room fall down? We don't know the answer." However, he pointed out that uterine cancer is highly detectable. "A woman can just have a hysterectomy." Critics of tamoxifen as prevention point out that because women in clinical trials are followed closely, their uterine cancers would be detected early. Outside a trial, women are not tracked with the same rigor, therefore uterine cancers could go undetected for a long time. So, based on this information, do you take the drug or not?

Hormone replacement therapy—does it cause cancer? Yes. No. Does it prevent heart disease? Yes. No. A senior doctor at the University of Toronto comments drily: "One reassuring thing is that if two studies flatly disagree, then you can be sure that neither is the truth."

There has been a steady flip-flop on mammography: some researchers, physicians, and large American cancer agencies support screening mammography for all women over the age of forty; others, including Canadian agencies, say no, only at age fifty. Some say mammography *causes* cancer, even the current machines with low-dose radiation; Dr. Rosalie Bertell points out that low-dose is totally relative anyway, that a four-film mammogram subjects the breast to a dosage of radiation one thousand times the strength of a chest X-ray, and that breast tissue is particularly vulnerable to radiation damage. "It's close enough to break the DNA," she points out. Others claim it's the best method we have for early detection, a claim countered by those who say that for a tumor to be big enough to be detectable by a mammogram, it would have to have been growing for seven or eight years already. The debate doesn't stop there. Some argue that early detection—through mammography—is finding cancers that probably would never have developed in the woman's lifetime and therefore should have been left alone. And still others say that the pressure of a mammogram is such that it can rupture small tumors, scattering cancer cells through the breast like seeds on fertile ground.

In the world of alternative cancer treatment, "experts" also contradict, argue, and deny each other. At the Tijuana cancer clinics, one says that pure dietary approaches are the only way; another says, absolutely not, you must use supplements. One claims that carrot juice is the elixir of life, the only way to beat cancer; another snorts in derision and forbids carrots in any form at his clinic because they are full of sugar.

How to decide? You struggle your way through information overload, you read the articles and books, you surf the Net, you sort it all out, and go to your doctors—only to get caught in the medical crossfire between experts who disagree, not in general, but on your specific case.

That's what happened to Rachel (not her real name), who had a non-aggressive breast cancer and a lumpectomy to remove it. Her doctor told her that she did not need adjuvant therapy. Five years later, it came back in the same breast; she had another lumpectomy, radiation treatments, and this time started taking tamoxifen. Then she fell into that gap left when science outstrips medicine, a gap that seems to fill up with conjecture. Genetic testing now can tell a woman about her probable risks in developing breast cancer either for the first time or again. Apparently not totally accurately, but still, the risk is identified. But then what? A gulf is opened up between the knowledge that she has the breast cancer gene and the ability to do anything about it. Preventive genetic therapy is still years away. (Dr. Steven Narod, associate professor in the Faculty of Medicine at the University of Toronto and chair of breast cancer research at Women's College Hospital, Toronto, doubts it will *ever* happen. It is not simply going in and altering the offending gene, as some media reports suggest; it is, rather, a highly complex tinkering which most women, high-risk or not, would not volunteer to be involved in. "Gene therapy means that if the gene is not working—a mutation—you replace the gene. It's very theoretical. I wouldn't get too excited about that. There are some studies on animals, some studies on different diseases, but there's no evidence yet that it is going to be effective on cancer. I mean it might be, but there is no clear path. . . . To use gene therapy on healthy women who have the gene defect to try and prevent cancer, I cannot see that study ever happening."

Any other preventive therapies currently available to a woman with the breast cancer gene are pretty grim. When testing indicated that Rachel has the breast cancer gene, she sought advice from two different doctors, both eminent in the field of breast cancer treatment and genetics.

The first doctor told Rachel that she had a 50 to 60 percent risk of developing a new primary breast cancer because of the gene. The second doctor told her that she had a 25 to 30 percent risk of developing a new primary.

A published source (Markman 1997) reports the lifetime risk of breast cancer for women with the BRCA-1 abnormality is approximately 85 percent, with a 60 percent prevalence before age fifty, but that only between 5 and 10 percent of women with breast cancer have the gene.

Both of Rachel's doctors agreed that having a prophylactic bilateral mastectomy would reduce her risk by 90 percent.

Rachel was drowning in a statistical quagmire.

First, she is presented with a 50 percent range of disagreement about her risk of developing breast cancer again. This gap yawns at her feet as she tries to make a decision that will have enormous consequences for every aspect of her life. Prophylactic bilateral mastectomy is the cutting off of both breasts to remove a possible site for a breast cancer to grow. And anyway, would this be tantamount to slamming the barn door after the horse has bolted? Some experts say that once a tumor in the breast is detectable, it has already spread, it is already a systemic disease. There is a growing school of thought that it is far less to do with treatment than with the immune system of the host whether it will develop into a full-blown metastasis.

Second, she is told that her risk of recurrence will be reduced by 90 percent if she opts to go this route. Sounds reassuring. But look again. That is 90 percent of either 50 percent or 25 percent of the original risk. An actuarial analysis of all the stats indicates that her risk could be much lower than it first appears. Then she is told that, at age sixty, a woman with the breast cancer gene has the same risk of developing the disease as does a woman without. She might also read about a more recent theory positing that breast cancer is really three separate diseases, and comes in three speeds: the mean type that spreads so quickly that current technology cannot detect or treat it; the second that is slower but will still spread within five or ten years; and a third type that takes even longer to spread, if it spreads at all. Rachel's first cancers were "non-aggressive." Could this mean that even if she did develop breast cancer again, it could be the languorous non-spreading type, making the sacrifice of both breasts unnecessary? Not really, it appears, because there is no certainty that if she did have a recurrence it would be the same type of cancer.

Now, in this new world of information-empowering opportunities, Rachel is told to decide what she wants to do, basing that decision on these conflicting data and theories. Let us know; now off you go.

The surgery is extensive. If Rachel chooses the mastectomies, she will have reconstruction. Marvellous things can be done with reconstructive surgery. A friend who had a mastectomy for breast cancer, a second mastectomy for prophylactic reasons, and then reconstruction, is understandably proud of her "amazing new boobs, "as she calls them. Beautifully shaped, with tattooed nipples, they have been constructed from her own flesh taken from the belly. The scarring is minimal, despite the amount of cutting. "The tattoos are fading," she says matter-of-factly. "I've got to go and have them redone." It used to be that in some mastectomies the nerves leading to the nipples could be preserved. A chilling sentence in a recent study on this procedure states that this is not a viable option anymore. That's all it says, no reason given why the procedure isn't viable.

But wait. At the First World Breast Cancer Conference, held in Kingston, Ontario in 1997, Dr. Narod spoke about the breast cancer gene and possible treatments for women to consider. He mentioned prophylactic chemotherapy. Could Rachel choose that instead? She could, but it still doesn't get her out of the world of ifs and maybes. Prophylactic chemotherapy in this instance is tamoxifen. She has already been taking it for five years, and there is controversy about both its safety and its efficacy after the five-year mark.

So what does she do? Does she continue to take tamoxifen, despite the risks? Does she have the surgery? Or does she do nothing? Does she abandon trying to make an "informed" decision and trust her instincts? However she arrives at her decision, she must live with the responsibility of making it, because with the new empowerment of the patient (in some cases, not even a patient yet, but a person who is told by genetic scientists that she probably soon will be) comes the burden of choice.

While Rachel struggled with her decision, one of the original doctors who had suggested she consider a prophylactic mastectomy now was saying, Well, hold on, maybe this isn't the route to take. New studies not yet published seem to indicate another possibility. It seems that the problem may lie in the way women respond to estrogen. It appears that for women with the breast cancer gene, estrogen encourages the growth of cancer cells at a ferocious rate. A more successful treatment may be an oophorectomy to remove the ovaries as the main source of estrogen. Dr. Narod says this isn't a new idea, that a major study on the efficacy of oophorectomies in the treatment of breast cancer was published in 1896. What goes around, comes around, but with the added knowledge this time of the genetic factor.

In the midst of all this, Rachel was forced to "take control" in a completely unexpected way. Because Rachel is part of a study of women with high risk for breast cancer, and she is closely tracked. When she asked about an enlarged lymph node, one of the study doctors suggested an ultrasound, which indicated nothing amiss. Rachel was given a choice: wait and watch it for six months, or have a core biopsy (in which a largish needle with a hollow core is used to extract cells). With Rachel's history that was an easy decision. She opted for the biopsy. Her own oncologist told her a few days later that he would never have suggested a core biopsy under the circumstances. But Rachel is not a medical practitioner, so she had no idea that such a procedure is not recommended when there is only a suspicion that there might be cancer. "When a woman goes into a study, she's sort of on loan to other doctors. I should have been told to discuss this procedure with my own oncologist. But I wasn't." Rachel was being asked to make a decision without being given the facts to support it.

Notwithstanding, the biopsy results came back positive and Rachel was hurled back into the nightmare. Within three weeks she had surgery to remove all the lymph nodes in her shoulder. And no cancer was found in any of them. How could that be? No one seemed to know. Was it possible that the biopsied cells had been contaminated in the lab? One other woman had been diagnosed with breast cancer the same day; perhaps her cells had somehow been mixed in with Rachel's, the same forceps used to transfer the cells, or the same slide. DNA testing was the way to find out.

"At this point," Rachel says, "I felt like I was driving a wild animal. It took a week for them to decide where to send the cell tissue for testing. After two more weeks I was told, 'Oh yes, we got the results yesterday but they were unsuccessful. The tissue sample was too small.' After three weeks of waiting, and now this. I couldn't believe it. Much of what happened from then on was at my suggestion. Throughout this whole process I kept phoning people, leaving messages. . . ." In effect, Rachel became her own care coordinator.

She had already tracked the pathologist to his lab-lair, discussed her case directly with him, and walked the corridors of at least three hospitals to seek out the various doctors involved in her cancer care; only when she suggested that the cells be sent to a forensic lab equipped to deal with smaller samples did the hospital take that step. In the meantime, she put her life on hold.

Her frustration was reaching boiling point, fueled by the hospitals' laconic responses to her attempts to find out if she actually had cancer again or if she had just undergone an invasive surgery for nothing. Her disposition was not improved by advice from her doctor that she should not lift heavy parcels with the arm with no lymph nodes, nor have blood drawn from it. She had no lymph nodes in her other arm either; they had been removed in her previous surgery. "Guess what," she snapped, "I've only got two arms."

In desperation she tried to make them see her point. All she wanted was to find out the status of her health, to find out if she was back in that other place, the world of the sick, the world of chemotherapy or radiation. "This is important to me," she told them. "It's also important to you."

The veiled threat seems to have clarified their focus, because very soon after, she was contacted by an administrator from one of the hospitals who offered to be her point person. She commiserated with Rachel, saying that she recognized how difficult it was for her to be dealing with so many different people. "She was very nice," Rachel says. And very guileless. "When I asked her exactly what she did in administration, she said, 'risk management.'" The hospital's, not Rachel's. A senior pathologist called her from Europe to assure her that he was keeping tabs on her case. His apparent concern was undermined by the timing of his call—three o'clock in the morning. "I was speechless," Rachel says. "He knew less about my case than I did. He didn't apologize for waking us, just said that he wanted me to know that he was staying involved. I lay awake seething for the next three hours. That morning I decided to call a lawyer. It's ironic, this is the last thing I wanted to do. I just wanted to know about my health. I just wanted to collaborate, to try to improve the process, to make sure this didn't happen to anyone else. But they have to learn, they have to re-evaluate their system."

There is certainly something wrong with this picture. Taking control is a great idea, but not when you're steering in a fog, falling down knowledge gaps, swirling in a syrup of conflicting information, misled by questionable test results, and getting help from the medical bureaucracy only when there's a risk you'll get litigious.

Somewhere, at some point in treatment, you will probably find yourself asking many of the same questions, encountering the same non-answers as Edwina and Rachel. It is the nature of the beast you are fighting; scientists try and contain it in nets of statistics and probabilities; oncologists try and poison it; radiologists burn it; surgeons carve it out; immunologists boost the body's ability to withstand its attacks; geneticists try and track it to its lair; and still it can shrug them all off. It still fools us with its unpredictable behavior, savaging one person to death, but sparing another after just a bite or two. Until we can know what it will do every time, many of our questions will continue to have no answers.

15
The Man Who Killed Starfish

Just as cancer enters lives in a variety of ways, so it leaves. After years in the world of cancer, you may wake one morning and NOT think of cancer. You may have slowly slipped the bounds of the disease, hardly realizing that you are almost back in your pre-cancer life, or reborn into a post-cancer one. Or cancer may leave as suddenly as it came, called by some a "spontaneous remission," by others a miracle, by others an assurance that you never had cancer in the first place.

Or cancer may not leave at all, but take its host into death, slowly, inexorably, by the book—treading the path laid down by statistics—or swiftly, with no warning even that it existed. The patient may accept with resignation, going gently into that good night with understanding and gratitude for the life lived; or he or she may go fighting every inch of the way, resisting death and the unknown.

Annabel Brown and Don Butterworth both went to the IAT Clinic after being diagnosed with mesothelioma. Neither lived longer than the statistical probability of survival of eleven months after diagnosis.

Braxton Colley was diagnosed with the same cancer in 1993. Seven years later, he is doing well. Earl Briscoe has been living with mesothelioma for fourteen years after his diagnosis.

Eleanor Britton went back to Scotland from the IAT Clinic for Christmas. Her doubting oncologist was amazed and delighted. He now had a "skeptical interest in the clinic."

She and her husband, Bill, held a big party on Hogmanay— "A hundred friends all came to see Eleanor, to congratulate her, all those people who had expected never to see her again, they were glad to have been proven wrong. They all came across the New Year threshold . . . along with their germs."

The "first footer" who should have brought them luck for the New Year must have gone to someone else's house. Eleanor got flu, the usual Scottish winter affliction. She couldn't get rid of it; she was listless and tired. Finally Bill phoned the IAT Clinic: "I asked if we should come back earlier than scheduled for her tune-up visit? They said 'Yes, absolutely, right away.' We should have come back the day she got flu."

The "jags" had been bolstering an immune system already stressed and weakened by cancer. "She had nothing left over to fight off anything else."

Eleanor never really recovered from this setback. She died on September 9, 1996, more than a year after starting at the IAT Clinic.

Earl Kruger fought hard to beat his lung cancer. So did his wife, Leslye, supporting him in the search for a treatment that would slow or arrest the disease. But the tumors grew—much more slowly than they had been told they would be by oncologists in mainstream hospitals, but nevertheless continuing to expand. Earl died two years after diagnosis, peacefully, knowing that he had done all he could.

Diane Loader died one month short of two years after her diagnosis of lung cancer. On the IAT treatment she had lived more than a year longer than her prognosis at the Montreal hospital where she had been diagnosed. She lived well and symptom-free until the last weeks of her life. She was in hospital for less than three days before she died. One of her last requests was that her husband bring her a Bailey's, the drink that they had enjoyed together for years. She preferred that to morphine, which she rejected after one injection.

Barbara Paul died within six months of the detection of metastatic breast cancer. Her IAT serum did not slow the disease.

David Wieting came to the clinic with liver cancer, hepatitis C, and the probability of only a few more months of life. He died a year later, not of the cancer but of hepatitis C.

Theresa Tufaro is well and thriving, ten years after discovery of the malignant tumor that had pushed her heart aside and flattened a lung.

Faye Pennington returns to the IAT Clinic every year for a tune-up seventeen years after being told that her lymphoma was out of control and would kill her within months.

Sue Deiner, Helene Greenstein, and Marcia Frank all continue on the IAT serum which keeps their cancer at bay.

Woolly Setteducato arrived at the IAT Clinic in April 1994 following surgical removal of a tumor and twenty-six nodes, a second surgery to remove his stomach, and the whispered advice from a nurse in the recovery room, "Don't let them give you chemotherapy." He was seventy-one years old with a prognosis of less than six months. He lived another five years, mostly pain-free, a life full of zest and humor—and hope, which he managed to instill in every other cancer patient he met.

Sue McPherson survived two years beyond her prognosis of three months. She died in September 1999.

Edwina Smith uses chemotherapy, a vaccine, and a powerful determination to fight her cancer. She buys back chunks of her life by giving up equal chunks to the chemo. She has been almost eight years in the cancer lists.

From these cases, can a statistical analysis be derived? No. At least not a truthful one. You could, depending on your biases, assign each to a specific category—miracles, spontaneous remissions, proof of treatment success, proof of treatment failure—do a statistical summary, and then publish the results . . . which would immediately be challenged by someone else who had analyzed the same cases and come up with a different conclusion. Ultimately, each case is just that, one case, one person struggling with his or her brand of cancer. And if you have cancer, the people you want to hear about are the miracles, the spontaneous remissions, the successes, the ones who have survived their disease for months or years longer than their prognosis, no matter how. These are the comforts in a long night, because they provide part of the skein of hope, so important against a disease that has us on the ropes.

After more than four years of research; of reading, listening, questioning; of interviewing hundreds of patients; of talking to doctors in both the alternative and the conventional worlds; of trying to separate the hype from the honest reporting, the vested interests from the altruistic interests; of willing myself to find at least some answers—I find myself back at the beginning. The questions remain, the debates, the controversies, the fights, and the uncertainties, and I am sad for everyone who must try and make sense of such a world, not as an intellectual challenge, but as one of personal survival. It is a world of sound and fury, cries and whispers, posturings and pain. For all of us who have been alone in the night, one on one with our cancer and our fears, ultimately all of it is just words. Yes, there are good doctors and bad doctors, good research, bad research, and biased research; there are media breakthroughs that are not breakthroughs at all, but headlines for a slow news day; there is real progress, and there are blind alleys; there is duplicity and in-fighting in places of power; there is also honesty and a genuine attempt to find answers; there is protectionism for good and bad reasons; there are fights over market share; there are cover-ups and courageous whistle-blowers who expose them. I guess, until cancer is eradicated from this earth, it will continue to be so, because it is not just a disease, it is an industry, a battlefield, a state of mind. Until it is exterminated, as smallpox was officially in June 1999 when the last two specimens were ceremoniously destroyed—until then, cancer in all its guises will rule. Until then, for everyone who has been touched by it, gently or with withering violence, it is, finally, a battle fought alone.

For northerners in the tropics, Christmas seems a long way away, despite the colored lights, the fake evergreens decorated with all the traditional stuff. Carols play in every store. Few of the IAT patients will be going home. Some will have family join them. One woman's husband leaves on December 12 to get things straightened out at home. "I used to have a business there," he muses. It's a whole other world, distant and so much less important than this one. He will bring their kids back for Christmas with their mother.

Patients will go out for special dinners, perhaps at the favorite restaurant in Port Lucaya, Luciano's, overlooking the marina, where there will be a soft, warm breeze off the ocean, candlelight, and fine food. What more could one ask? Well, along with the grouper and garlic butter, you could ask that your cancer disappear, that you could go into rewind to the days before diagnosis, and take another route that detours the tests, the waiting rooms, the devastating words, "You have cancer," the painful surgery, the nauseating chemo, the difficult, gut-wrenching decisions, the despair, the fear—a route that brings you instead to this fine island as a tourist, on vacation, like everyone else in the restaurant or on the beach. Well, nearly everyone.

The man in the singlet and baseball cap didn't join the IAT patients and their families for any festivities. He was rarely seen at the clinic. He just kept killing starfish. Kneeling at the edge of the surf, he scooped and sliced at the innards like a mad surgeon. The sun glinted off the knife as it scraped the cavity, keeping the tentacles intact. The bowl in front of him, balanced on an altar of driftwood, was filling up with starfish, sacrificed to his pain and desperate prayers to save his son. He didn't look up from his task when his wife came and sat at the water's edge beside him. She watched the slicing knife, wordless. Their son stood, his thin, delicate body a black silhouette etched against the flashing sundrench of the sea. The mother, father, and son, a triptych family, frozen for a moment in the December sun on a Bahamas beach. Not a star in sight. No shepherds kneeling, no wise men with answers, but still a hard time of it. And the sound of tearing flesh from bone. The boy's cancer was not responding to treatment. It was consuming his frail body. It was consuming his family.

A roil of cloud sent a shadow across the sand, a cold wind stirred the shivering sunbathers. They gathered their chairs, their beach bags, their vacation paraphernalia, and headed to the beach bar for happy hour. The father stayed on the shore, raging, raging at the dying of the light.

Every afternoon, all that week, the man came to the edge of the sea in the afternoon, knelt, and killed starfish. The boy did not come again.

Bibliography

Altman, Roberta, and Michael J. Sarg, M.D. (1992). *The Cancer Dictionary*. New York: Facts on File Inc.

American Biologies. (n.d.) "There are no 'Matching Cases' and these are NOT 400 'Kinds' or 'Types' of Cancer." Information sheet. Tijuana: America Biologies.

Anderson, Alan, Jr. (1974). "The Politics of Cancer: How Do You Get the Medical Establishment to Listen?" *New York Magazine*. (29 July).

Annals of Internal Medicine. (1996). "Bone Marrow Transplantation." 625–33.

Antman, Blum, et al. (1980). "Multimodality Therapy for Malignant Mesothelioma Based on a Study of Natural History." *American Journal of Medicine* vol. 68 (March).

Bailar, John C. III, and Heather L. Gornik. (1997). "Cancer Undefeated." *New England Journal of Medicine* vol. 336, no. 22.

Beauregard, Karen M., Susan K. Drilea, and Jessica P. Vistnes. (1996). "The Uninsured in America: 1996." MEPS Highlight from the *Medical Expenditure Panel Survey of the Agency of Health Care Policy and Research*. Web site: *http://www.meps.ahcpr.gov/highlit/mephihg1*.

Beinfield, Harriet, and Malcolm S. Beinfield. (1997). "Revisiting Accepted Wisdom in the Management of Breast Cancer." *Alternative Therapies* vol. 3, no. 5 (September).

Bird, Christopher. (1990). *The Galileo of the Microscope: The Life and Trials of Gaston Naessens*. St. Lambert, Quebec: Les Presses de l'Université de la Personne Inc.

Braverman, Albert, M.D. (1991). "Medical Oncology in the 1990s." *The Lancet* 337: 901–02.

Brenner, David J., and Eric J. Hall. (1996). *Making the Radiation Therapy Decision.* Los Angeles: RGA Publishing Group (Lowell House).

Broyard, Anatole. (1992). *Intoxicated by My Illness.* New York: Clarkson Potter.

Buckman, Robert. (1996). *What You Really Need to Know About Cancer.* Toronto: Key Porter Books. [1995]. (Page references are to the London Macmillan edition [1996]).

———, and Karl Sabbach. (1995). *Magic or Medicine? An Investigation of Healing and Healers.* New York: Prometheus Books.

Bujold, Isabelle. (1996). "Diagnosis and Treatment: Taxotere." *Revue du REIQCS* (English version) vol. 1, no. 2 (Spring).

Canadian Breast Cancer Network (CBCN). (1998). *Network News: The National Network and Voice of Breast Cancer Survivors.* Newsletter. Ottawa: CBCN.

Canadian Broadcasting Corporation (CBC). (1997). *Market Place*: "At What Price?" Transcript. (November 11).

———. Canadian Broadcasting Corporation (CBC). (1999). *Market Place*: "False Hope in a Mexican Cancer Clinic." Transcript. (January 19).

Canadian Medical Association. (1998). "A Patient's Guide to Choosing Unconventional Therapies." *Canadian Medical Association Journal* vol. 158, no. 9.

Cancer Control Society (CCS). (n.d.). "The Association Story." Los Angeles: CCS.

Cassileth, Barrie J., et al. (1991). "Survival and Quality of Life Among Patients Receiving Unproven as Compared with Conventional Cancer Therapy." *New England Journal of Medicine* vol. 324, no. 17 (April 25).

CDC (Centers for Disease Control). "Recommendations for Protection Against Viral Hepatitis." *Annals of Internal Medicine* 103: 391–402.

———. Web site. (1999). *National Census on Health Statistics: Fastats. www.cdc.gov/nchswww/fastats/cancer.*

Centre for Intergrated Healing. (1999). "Blue Book," Vancouver: Centre for Integrated Healing, Suite 200–1330 West 8th Avenue, Vancouver BC, V6H 4A6

The Choice. (1998). Official Publication of the Committee for Freedom of Choice in Medicine, Inc. (Chula Vista, Calif.). vol. 24, no. 1.

Chopra, Deepak. (1989). *Quantum Healing. Exploring the Frontiers of Mind Body Medicine.* New York: Bantam Books.

Clement, John; Lawrence Burton; and Gerald N. Lampe. "Peritoneal Mesothelioma." *Quantum Medicine* vol. 1, no. 1 (January 1988. Updated by J. Clements, 1998.)

Collinge, William. (1996). *The American Holistic Health Association Complete Guide to Alternative Medicine*. New York: Warner Books.

COSE. (1995). Centre d'Orthobiologie Somatidienne de l'Estrie Inc. Letter from Kim Lalancette to author, July 7. (Telephone confirmation with COSE staff, October 1999.)

Cottman, Evans W., with Wyatt Blassingame. (1963). *Out-Island Doctor*. London: Hodder & Stoughton.

de Bernières, Louis. (1995). *Captain Corelli's Mandolin*. London: Mandarin Paperbacks, Minerva Edition.

Donsbach, Kurt W., and H. Rudolph Alsleban. (1993). *Wholistic Cancer Therapy*. The Rockland Corporation; tel: 1-800-421-7310.

Dooling, Richard. (1992). *Critical Care*. New York: Picador.

Drum, David. (1998). *Making the Chemotherapy Decision*. Newly revised. 2nd ed. Los Angeles: RGA Publishing Group (Lowell House).

Elias, Thomas D. (1997). *The Burzynski Breakthrough: The Century's Most Promising Cancer Treatment and the Government's Campaign to Squelch It*. Los Angeles: General Publishing Group.

Epstein, Samuel S. (1998). *The Politics of Cancer Revisited*. Fremount Center, N.Y.: East Ridge Press.

Firth, Matthew, James Brophy, and Margaret Keith. (1997). *Workplace Roulette: Gambling with Cancer*. Toronto: Between the Lines.

Fisher, Bernard, and James Dignam. (1997). "Recent Findings from Three NSABP Clinical Trials Evaluating Systemic Adjuvant Therapy in Patients with Primary Breast Cancer and Negative Axillary Nodes." In Sydney E. Salmon, ed., *Adjuvant Therapy of Cancer* VIII. Proceedings of the Eighth International Conference on the Adjuvant Therapy of Cancer, Scotsdale, Arizona, March 1996. Philadelphia, New York: Lippincott/Raven.

Fist, Stewart. (1999). *Reporting Scientific Research*. Abstract. Program of World Conference on Breast Cancer, July 1999, Ottawa.

Flitter, Marc, M.D. (1997). *Judith's Pavilion: The Haunting Memories of a Neurosurgeon*. South Royalton, Vermont: Steerforth Press.

Fonfa, Ann E. (1998). Opening Statement to the U.S. Government Reform and Oversight Committee: Hearings. (February 4). Reprinted at web site: *www.ralphmoss.com/fonfa1.html*

————. (n.d.). *Outline of a Consumer's Guide of Alternative Medicine (for Cancer Patients)*. Unpublished. Available from author, 28 West 38th Street, Suite 12E, New York, NY 10018; tel: (212) 869-0139; e-mail: Ann Fonfa@aol.com

Fugh-Berman, Adriane. (1999a). "Harvard Survey of Alternative Medicine Use Updated." *Alternative Therapies in Women's Health* vol. 1, no. 2 (January).

————. (1999b). "Complementary Therapies and Breast Cancer." *Alternative Therapies in Women's Health* vol. 1, no. 5 (April).

Glasser, Ronald J. (1998) "The Doctor Is Not In," *Harper's* (March).

Globe and Mail. (1998a). "Study Can't Prove Tamoxifen Prevents Cancer." July 10.

————. (1998b). "Health Activists to Seek 'Asylum' in Canada." November 17.

GMDS *96. (1998). "The Controversy About the Association Between Sunscreen Use and Malignant Melanoma: Results of a Multicenter EORTC Case-Control Study." Website: Krebserrankungen. http://www.meb.uni-bon

Green, Daniel M., and Giulio J. D'Angio, eds. (1992). *Late Effects of Treatment for Childhood Cancer.* In series *Current Clinical Oncology.* New York: Wiley-Liss.

Green, Saul. (1993). "Immunoaugmentative Therapy: An Unproven Cancer Treatment." *Journal of the American Medical Association* vol. 270, no. 14 (October 13).

Groopman, Jerome, M.D. (1997). *The Measure of Our Days.* New York: Viking Penguin.

Hitchens, Christopher. (1998). "Bitter Medicine." *Vanity Fair* (August).

Hoy, Claire. (1995). *The Truth About Breast Cancer.* Toronto: Stoddart Publishing Company.

Hubbell, F. Allen, M.D.; Sheldon Greenfield, M.D.; Judy L. Tyler, M.P.H., et al. (1985). "The Impact of Routine Admission Chest X-ray Films on Patient Care." *New England Journal of Medicine* vol. 312, no. 4.

Junger, Sebastian. (1997). *The Perfect Storm: A True Story of Men Against the Sea.* New York: W.W. Norton & Company.

Kaegi, Elizabeth. (1998). "Unconventional Therapies for Cancer: 1. Essiac; 2. Green Tea; 3. Iscador; 4. Hydrazine sulfate; 5. Vitamins A, C and E; 6. 714-X." Reprinted from *Canadian Medical Association Journal* vol. 158, nos. 7–12.

Kaplan, Sheila, and Shannon Brownlee. (1999). "Dying for a Cure," *U.S. News and World Report.* (October 11).

Keizer, Bert. (1996). *Dancing with Mister D: Notes on Life and Death.* London: Doubleday, Transworld Publishers.

Krakoff, Irwin H., M.D. (1996). "Systemic Treatment of Cancer" CA—*A Cancer Journal for Clinicians* vol. 46, no. 3 (May/June).

Kübler-Ross, Elisabeth. (1997). *The Wheel of Life: A Memoir of Living and Dying.* New York: Scribner.

Lau, Andree. (1999). "The Hope and the Hype of Cancer Vaccines." *Catalyst* (January).

Manner, Harold W. (1989). *The Death of Cancer.* San Ysidro: Metabolic Research Foundation.

Markman, Maurie, M.D. (1997). *Basic Cancer Medicine.* Philadelphia: W.B. Saunders.

Maser, Michael. (1999). "Exploring the Alternatives in Cancer Treatment," *The Georgia Strait.* (August 26-September 2).

Medical Research Council, Canada. (1978). *Ethical Considerations in Research Involving Human Subjects.* Report No. 6. Ottawa.

Molloy, Dr. William. (1993). *Vital Choices: Life, Death and the Health Care Crisis.* Toronto: Penguin Books.

Moss, Ralph W. (1992). *Cancer Therapy: The Independent Consumer's Guide to Non-Toxic Treatment and Prevention.* New York: Equinox Press.

———. (1994). *The Cancer Chronicles.* Vol. 5, nos. 5-6 (November-December).

———. (1995). *Questioning Chemotherapy.* New York: Equinox Press.

———. (1996). *The Cancer Industry.* New updated ed. New York: Equinox Press.

National Bone Marrow Transplant Link. (1999). "How Much Does a Bone Marrow Transplant Typically Cost?" Web site: *http://comnet.org/nbontlink/cost*

National Cancer Institute of Canada. (1999). *Canadian Cancer Statistics 1999.*

National Cancer Institute (U.S.). (1999). National Institutes of Health Press Releases. Web site: *rex.nci.nih.gov*

National Post. (1999) "Breakthrough in Breast Cancer Treatment." April 13.

Nuland, Sherwin B. (1995). *Doctors: The Biography of Medicine.* 2nd ed. New York: Vintage Books.

———. (1988). *How We Live.* New York: Vintage Books.

Null, Gary. (1987). "You Are the Victim." *Penthouse.* No. 16 in a series "Medical Genocide" (October).

———, and Leonard Steinman. (1986). "The Vendetta Against Dr. Burton." *Penthouse.* No. 7 in a series "Medical Genocide" (March).

O'Hara, Jane. (1998). "Whistle-Blower." *Maclean's* (November 16).

Ontario Breast Cancer Information Exchange Project (OBCIEP) (under the federal Breast Cancer Initiative). (1994). *A Guide to Unconventional Cancer Therapies.* Toronto: OBCIEP.

———. (n.d.). *Breast Cancer Info Exchange.* Toronto: OBCIEP.

Ottawa Citizen. (1996). "The Doctor Is Online." April 29.

———. (1998a). "LSD Experiments 'Good Research Back Then.'" July 10.

———. (1998b). "Cancer Doctor a Superstar." June 8.

———. (1998c). "When Professionalism Weakens Civility." John Polanyis address to the M.D. graduates at the University of Toronto's Faculty of Medicine, June 1998. July 16.

———. (1999a). "Cancer Researchers Optimistic." February 8.

———. (1999). Editorial. "Bad Medicine." July 29.

Patterson, James T. (1987). *The Dread Disease: Cancer and Modern American Culture*. Cambridge, Mass: Harvard University Press.

Paulsen, Monte. (1994). "The Cancer Business." *Mother Jones* (May/June).

Pearson, Hugh. (1995). "Editorial: The Need to Liberate Physicians to Practice Complementary Medicine." *Journal of Orthomolecular Medicine* vol. 10, nos. 3 & 4.

Pelton, Ross, and Lee Overholser. (1994). *Alternatives in Cancer Therapy: The Complete Guide to Non-Traditional Treatments*. New York: Simon & Schuster (A Fireside Book).

Peterkin, Allan D. (1998). *Staying Human During Residency Training*. 2nd ed. Toronto: University of Toronto Press.

Porter, Roy. (1997a). *The Greatest Benefit to Mankind: A Medical History of Humanity*. New York: W.W. Norton.

———. ed. (1997b). *Medicine: A History of Healing*. New York: The Marlowe Company.

Price, Reynolds. (1995). *A Whole New Life: An Illness and a Healing*. New York: Penguin Group/Plume.

Proctor, Robert N. (1995). *Cancer Wars: How Politics Shapes What We Know and Don't Know About Cancer*. New York: Basic Books.

Richards, V. (1972). *Cancer, The Wayward Cell: Its Origins, Nature, and Treatment*. Berkeley: University of California Press.

Roberts, Paul William. (1992). "Blood Feud." *Saturday Night* (December).

Rosenfeld, Isadore, M.D. (1996). *Dr. Rosenfeld's Guide to Alternative Medicine: What Works, What Doesn't—And What's Right for You*. New York: Random House.

Roueché, Berton. (1996). *The Man Who Grew Two Breasts and Other True Tales of Medical Detection*. New York: Truman Talley Books/Plume.

Siegal, Bernie, M.D. (1986). *Love, Medicine and Miracles*. New York: Harper & Row.

———. (1989). *Peace Love and Healing: BodyMind Communication and the Path to Self-Healing: An Exploration*. New York: Harper & Row.

———. (1990). *Humor and Healing*. (Cassette). Boulder, Col.: Sounds True Recordings.

Spiegal, Maura, and Richard Tristman, eds. (1997). *The Grim Reader: Writings on Death, Dying, and Living On*. New York: Anchor Books, Doubleday.

Steingraber, Sandra. (1997). *Living Downstream. An Ecologist Looks at Cancer and the Environment*. New York: Addison-Wesley (A Merloyd Lawrence Book).

Stewart, Dr. L.A. (1998). "Postoperative Radiotherapy in Non-Small-Cell Lung Cancer: Systemic Review and Meta-analysis of Individual Patient Data from Nine Randomized Controlled Trials." *The Lancet* vol. 352.

Time Life Editors. (1996). *The Medical Advisor: The Complete Guide to Alternative and Conventional Treatment.* Time Life.

Trimble, Edward L. (1999). "The Role of Complementary and Alternative Medicine in the Detection and Treatment of Women's Cancers." Testimony at the Hearing before the House Committee on Government Reform (June 10). Web site: *http://waisgate.hhs.go*

United States. (1986). Congressional Hearing: A Hearing on the Immuno-Augmentative Therapy (IAT) of Dr. Lawrence Burton before Congressman Guy Molinari: Summary. New York (January 15).

———. (1999). President's Advisory Commission on Consumer Protection and Quality in the Health Care Industry. Final Report: *Improving Quality in a Changing Health Care Industry.* Web site: *http://waisgate.hhs.go*

Vialls, Joe. (1999). "The Ultimate Cancer Conspiracy: Vitamin B17 and Laetrile." Web site: *www.thuntek.net/sumaria*

Walters, Richard. (1993). *Options: The Alternative Cancer Therapy Book.* Garden City, N.Y.: Avery Publishing Group Inc.

Wente, Margaret. (1999a). "Consider Cancer's Charletons." *Globe and Mail* (July 8).

———. (1999b). "Truth Takes a Holiday." *Globe and Mail* (July 31).

Williams, Penelope. (1993). *That Other Place: A Personal Account of Breast Cancer.* Toronto: Dundurn Press.

Wilson, Benjamin, M.D. (1999). "The Rise and Fall of Laetrile." Web site: *www.quackwatch.com.*

Wright, Jane Riddle. (1985). *Diagnosis: Cancer; Prognosis: Life: The Story of Dr. Lawrence Burton and the Immunology Researching Centre.* Huntsville, Ala.: Albright & Co.

Index